JIMD Reports
Volume 45

Eva Morava
Editor-in-Chief

Matthias Baumgartner · Marc Patterson ·
Shamima Rahman · Johannes Zschocke
Editors

Verena Peters
Managing Editor

JIMD Reports
Volume 45

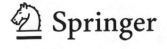 Springer

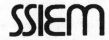

Editor-in-Chief
Eva Morava
Tulane University Medical School
New Orleans
Louisiana
USA

Editor
Matthias Baumgartner
Division of Metabolism & Children's Research
Centre
University Children's Hospital Zürich
Zürich
Switzerland

Editor
Marc Patterson
Division of Child and Adolescent Neurology
Mayo Clinic
Rochester
Minnesota
USA

Editor
Shamima Rahman
Clinical and Molecular Genetics Unit
UCL Institute of Child Health
London
UK

Editor
Johannes Zschocke
Division of Human Genetics
Medical University Innsbruck
Innsbruck
Austria

Managing Editor
Verena Peters
Center for Child and Adolescent Medicine
Heidelberg University Hospital
Heidelberg
Germany

ISSN 2192-8304   ISSN 2192-8312   (electronic)
JIMD Reports
ISBN 978-3-662-58646-4   ISBN 978-3-662-58647-1   (eBook)
https://doi.org/10.1007/978-3-662-58647-1

Contents

JIMD Reports
DOI 10.1007/8904_2018_130

RESEARCH REPORT

I-Cell Disease (Mucolipidosis II): A Case Series from a Tertiary Paediatric Centre Reviewing the Airway and Respiratory Consequences of the Disease

Rachel Edmiston · Stuart Wilkinson · Simon Jones · Karen Tylee · Alexander Broomfield · Iain A. Bruce

Received: 21 March 2018 / Revised: 18 July 2018 / Accepted: 25 July 2018 / Published online: 13 September 2018
© Society for the Study of Inborn Errors of Metabolism (SSIEM) 2018

Abstract *Background*: Inclusion cell disease (I-cell) is a rare autosomal recessive metabolic disease involving multiple organ systems, associated with a severely restricted life expectancy. No curative therapy is currently available, with management aimed at symptom palliation.

Methods: We present a retrospective, single-centre, case series of children referred to a tertiary paediatric metabolic service. The clinical presentation, demographics, genetics and natural history of the condition are investigated.

Results: Five patients with I-cell disease were referred over a 10-year period. All patients were born with dysmorphic features and had a family history of I-cell disease on further exploration. Phenotypic variation was seen within patients with the same genetic profile. Airway problems were common with 100% of the documented sleep oximetry studies suggesting sleep-disordered breathing. Of the two patients who had tracheal intubation anaesthetic difficulties we encountered, one required intra-operative reintubation, and one suffered a failed intubation with subsequent death. All five patients required oxygen therapy with the use of CPAP and BiPAP also seen. Feeding issues were almost universal with four of the five patients requiring nasogastric feeding. Four patients had died in the 10-year period with a mean life expectancy of 36 months. Cause of death for three of the four patients was respiratory failure.

Conclusions: Airway problems, including sleep-disordered breathing, were ubiquitous in this cohort of children. Any intervention requiring a general anaesthetic needs careful multidisciplinary consideration due to significant associated risks and possibly death. Management as a result is generally non-surgical and symptomatic. This case series demonstrates universal involvement of the airway and respiratory systems, an important consideration when selecting meaningful outcomes for future effectiveness studies of novel therapies.

Communicated by: Roberto Giugliani, MD, PhD

R. Edmiston (✉) · I. A. Bruce
Paediatric ENT Department, Royal Manchester Children's Hospital, Manchester University Hospitals NHS Foundation Trust, Manchester Academic Health Science Centre, Manchester, UK
e-mail: Rachel.edmiston@nhs.net; Iain.bruce@mft.nhs.uk

S. Wilkinson
Paediatric Respiratory Department, Royal Manchester Children's Hospital, Manchester University Hospitals NHS Foundation Trust, Manchester Academic Health Science Centre, Manchester, UK
e-mail: Stuart.wilkinson@mft.nhs.uk

S. Jones · K. Tylee · A. Broomfield
Willink Biochemical Genetics Unit, Manchester Centre for Genomic Medicine, St. Mary's Hospital, Manchester University Hospitals NHS Foundation Trust, Manchester Academic Health Science Centre, Manchester, UK
e-mail: Simon.jones@mft.nhs.uk; Karen.tylee@mft.nhs.uk; Alexander.broomfield@mft.nhs.uk

I. A. Bruce
Division of Infection, Immunity and Respiratory Medicine, Faculty of Biology, Medicine and Health, University of Manchester, Manchester, UK

Abbreviations

BiPAP	Bilevel positive airway pressure
CPAP	Continuous positive airway pressure
ECHO	Echocardiogram
LMA	Laryngeal mask airway
NGT	Nasogastric tube
ODI	Oxygen deprivation index
OSA	Obstructive sleep apnoea
PDA	Patent ductus arteriosus
PEG	Percutaneous endoscopic gastrostomy
SDB	Sleep-disordered breathing

Background

Inclusion-cell disease or I-cell disease (mucolipidosis II) is a rare autosomal recessive metabolic disease with a prevalence of 1 in 100,000–400,000. Patients present from birth with a severe skeletal dysplasia and profound short stature. Characteristic features include craniofacial abnormalities (enlarged skull, gingival hyperplasia, flat nasal bridge and macroglossia), musculoskeletal malformations (abnormally shaped vertebrae and ribs, hypoplastic epiphyses, bullet-shaped metacarpals) and severe cardiac and respiratory problems that result in early death usually between the fifth and seventh year of life (Wiesmann and Herschkowitz 1981).

The disease results from an intracellular deficiency of multiple lysosomal hydrolases leading to a complex storage phenotype. The primary defect has been found to be a deficiency of UDP-*N*-acetylglucosamine-1-phosphate transferase (GlcNAc-P transferase) activity (Mueller et al. 1983). Lack of this protein leads to abnormally glycosylated hydrolytic enzymes and a subsequent failure of trafficking of these enzymes to the lysosome with subsequent secretion into the extracellular compartment (Cathy et al. 2008).

Due to the multi-organ involvement, the management of I-cell patients requires a multidisciplinary team approach with paediatricians, geneticists, respiratory and cardiac physicians and otolaryngology surgeons all playing an important role. The progressive nature of this currently incurable disease necessitates appropriate parental support, with the ultimate objective being to optimize quality of life and palliation.

Despite airway sequelae being a large contributory factor in the morbidity associated with I-cell disease, little has been written reflecting the particular perspectives of respiratory and ENT specialists.

Methods and Inclusion Criteria

In this case series, we present our population of patients diagnosed with I-cell disease in the last 10 years and managed at our tertiary paediatric centre. We will review their genotypic and phenotypic differences to demonstrate key strategies that can be employed to aid in diagnosis and management. Our patient experience will be linked to a comprehensive literature search applied to EMBASE and MEDLINE with no limits using a medical subject headings (MeSH) search linking I-cell disease to ENT issues (Table 1).

I-cell disease is defined in multiple ways within current literature with a lot of crossover between other lysosomal

Table 1 MeSH headings

MeSH headings (combined with mucolipidosis II OR I-cell)	
Airway	Tonsils
Sleep apnoea	Adenoids
Sleep apnoea	Hearing
Sleep apnoea syndrome	Conductive hearing loss
Sleep apnoea syndrome	Sensorineural hearing loss
Airway obstruction	Otolaryngology
Obstructive sleep apnoea	Otorhinolaryngologic disease
Obstructive sleep apnoea	Tracheostomy
Snoring	Nasal polyps
Otitis media	Sinusitis
Otitis media with effusion	Rhinitis
Anaesthesia	Adenoidectomy
Anaesthetic	Tonsillectomy
	Deafness

storage diseases. Our diagnostic criteria for inclusion in this paper included:

- Characteristic clinical features
- Genetic mutations (GNPTAB gene)
- Plasma lysosomal enzyme levels

Patient records were reviewed including paper notes and electronic records.

Results

Baseline Data

Five patients met the inclusion criteria as stated above, three females and two males. At the time of data collection, only one patient was still alive aged 35 months (patient 5).

Patient 1 died aged 19 months, patient 2 died aged 4 months, patient 3 died aged 97 months, and patient 4 died aged 25 months (mean life expectancy = 36 months).

Cause of death was available for three of the patients. Patients 1 and 3 died of respiratory failure. Patient 4 had respiratory failure with a failed intubation at the end of life.

Diagnosis

Age at Diagnosis

The age of diagnosis varied significantly with patient 4 being diagnosed at 3 days and patient 3 being diagnosed at 44 weeks. Of note patient 3 was the older sibling of patient 4 facilitating earlier diagnosis, and patient 3 was the first family member to have a genetic condition, and as such a final diagnosis was slower to achieve.

Presenting Features (See Table 2)

All patients were born with dysmorphic features including micrognathia, gingival hypertrophy and retroglossia, and in the male children, hypospadias was common. Other features included talipes, polydactyly, perinatal fractures and chest wall asymmetry. See Fig. 1.

Ethnicity

Four of the five patients were British Pakistani, and one was a white Irish traveller (patient 5).

All patients had family members with I-cell disease with patients 1 and 2 and patients 3 and 4 being siblings. Parental consanguinity was present in patients 1–4. Patient 5 had multiple family members with I-cell disease including their paternal grandmother and two cousins.

Birth

Three of the five babies were born at term with one spontaneous delivery at 34 weeks and another elective caesarian section at 27 + 4 weeks. Only two of the patients had antenatal problems including intrauterine growth restriction in one and foetal tachycardia and oligohydramnios in another. One patient developed antenatal fractures secondary to hyperparathyroidism.

Genetics

Each family had a different genetic profile, and though siblings shared mutations, there were significant phenotypic variations in the presentation of the disease (see Table 2). Two genotypes were found with patients 1, 2 and 5 sharing the same variant and siblings (patient 3 and 4) sharing another. Genotypes seen in Irish travellers and British Pakistani patients tend to be shared and common to those ethnicities (Lynch et al. 2018). While these mutations (typically in homozygous form) tend to give rise to a severe phenotype, there exists considerable variability even within families.

Airway/Anaesthetic and Respiratory Issues

Sleep oximetry studies were only available for three of the five patients. All demonstrated sleep-disordered breathing (SDB) (defined as an oxygen deprivation index ODI 4%

Table 2 Patients genotype and phenotypic variations

Patient	Genotype	Presenting features	Main issues
1 (Female) (sibling of patient 2) **AAD: 8 weeks** **DOD: 11/4/13 (19 months)**	GNPTAB gene: homozygous c.3503_3504delTC	Dysmorphic features, poor swallow, talipes, polydactyly	Sleep-disordered breathing Long-term oxygen Nasogastric feeding
2 (Female) (sibling of patient 1) **AAD: 2 weeks** **DOD: 17/11/14 (4 months)**	GNPTAB gene: homozygous c.3503_3504delTC	Dysmorphic features, IUGR, hyperparathyroidism, skeletal demineralisation, vit D deficiency, chronic lung disease, dilated left ventricle	Long-term oxygen Nasogastric feeding
3 (Male) (sibling of patient 4) **AAD: 44 weeks** **DOD: 1/12/15 (97 months)**	GNPTAB gene: homozygous mutation c.1314_1315delTG	Dysmorphic features, micrognathia, hypospadias, gingival hypertrophy, retroglossia, chest wall asymmetry	Sleep-disordered breathing Nocturnal oxygen BiPAP Respiratory failure: (diagnosed age 26 months) Pulmonary hypertension Nasogastric feeding Otitis externa
4 (Female) (sibling of patient 3) **AAD: 3 days** **DOD: 24/11/17 (25 months)**	GNPTAB gene: homozygous mutation c.1314_1315delTG	Dysmorphic features, hyperparathyroidism, multiple fractures, talipes, thrombocytopenia	Long-term oxygen Nasogastric feeding
5 (Male) **AAD: 6 weeks**	GNPTAB gene: homozygous c.3503_3504delTC	Dysmorphic features, high bilirubin, galactosaemia	Sleep-disordered breathing Long-term oxygen Respiratory failure: (diagnosed age 9 months) Nasogastric feeding Inguinal hernias

Bold text indicates dates
AAD age at diagnosis, *DOD* date of death

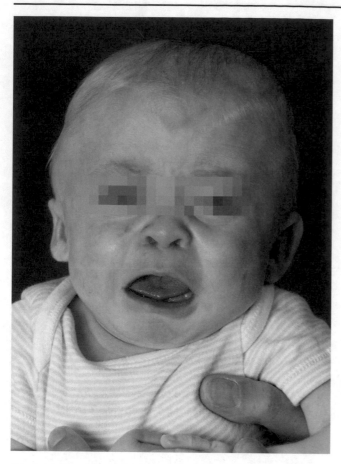

Fig. 1 Characteristic facial dysmorphism in a young child with I-cell disease

>3 events/h and median saturation of <85% equating to McGill criteria 3 or 4 (Brouillette et al. 2000) with 4% oxygen deprivation indices (ODI/h) levels ranging from 8.25 to 42.5 (see Table 3).

All patients required oxygen supplementation therapy. Data was absent for one patient, but three patients required constant long-term oxygen and one received nocturnal oxygen therapy. Starting age of oxygen therapy varied with one patient never coming off treatment from birth and one commencing therapy at 24 months. Median age of oxygen therapy commencement was 7 months.

Patients were defined as having type II respiratory failure if there was a documented PCO2 >50 mmHg (6.7 kPa). Three patients had gas measurements within the notes confirming this; however, only one patient required BiPAP (bilevel positive airway pressure) support via nasal non-invasive ventilation (NIV). The age of starting BiPAP support was 26 months, and it was required 24 h a day until they died aged 97 months. One patient received CPAP but only during an acute exacerbation over a 2 week period. Despite absent gas measurements in the patient records of the two other patients, they had a documented cause of death as respiratory failure.

Only one patient had general anaesthetic procedures performed both after their diagnosis. Their first procedure aged 4 months was for bilateral herniotomies for which they had an uncomplicated general anaesthetic with a grade 1 intubation. The second procedure (insertion of a ventriculoperitoneal shunt) at 31 months was performed as a result of communicating hydrocephalus resulting in vision loss. The initial anaesthetic technique was with the use of a nasopharyngeal and laryngeal mask airway (LMA). Using the technique described by Walker et al. (1997), a bronchoscope was introduced via the LMA to gain a view of the trachea. After the cords were sprayed with local anaesthetic, a guide wire was introduced through the bronchoscope port and the bronchoscope removed. An exchange catheter was then introduced over the wire to enable both the wire and LMA to be removed and endotracheal intubation to be performed over the exchange catheter. The tube placement was found to be very positional due to presumed tracheomalacia, and an uncomplicated tube change (increased size) was performed mid-procedure using a GlideScope with a grade 2 view. The patient was noted to ventilate better in a head-up and head-extended position.

Cardiac Issues

Within our group three of the five patients had abnormal findings on their echocardiograms. Patient 3 was the only patient to develop pulmonary hypertension and had specific treatment for this in the form of sildenafil, patient 2 demonstrated cardiomegaly on their ECHO, and patient 4 had a patent foramen ovale and PDA which closed spontaneously.

Feeding Issues

Only one patient managed oral intake as a primary means of nutrition. Patients 1–4 required nutritional supplementation via a nasogastric tube (NGT), and in all of these patients, multiple conversations were held as to the placement of a percutaneous endoscopic gastrostomy (PEG), but in all cases patients were deemed unfit for surgery. NGT feeding however was well tolerated in all these patients.

ENT Manifestations of Disease and Treatment

Although SDB was ubiquitous, none of our patients underwent airway surgery (adenotonsillectomy/tracheostomy) due to concerns about life-threatening airway complications during anaesthesia and in the event of post-adenotonsillectomy bleeding.

Table 3 Completed data set

	Patient 1	Patient 2	Patient 3	Patient 4	Patient 5
Gender	Female	Female	Male	Female	Male
Ethnic origin	Asian Pakistani	Asian Pakistani	Asian Pakistani	Asian Pakistani	White Irish (inc. traveller)
Birth	34 weeks gestation Normal delivery	27 + 4 weeks gestations Elective section	40 weeks gestation Emergency section	39 + 2 weeks gestation Emergency section	37 + 5 weeks gestation Normal delivery
Sleep-disordered breathing	Yes	Undocumented	Yes	Undocumented	Yes
	4% ODI/h: 13 Min sat: 62.6% Mean sat: 95% Age at test: 17 months		4% ODI/h: 8.25 Min sat: 71.8% Mean sat: 96% Age at test: 96 months		4% ODI/h: 42.5 Min sat: 77% Mean sat: 97% Age at test: 10 months
Oxygen therapy	Yes: long-term oxygen from 24 months	Yes: long-term oxygen from birth	Yes: nocturnal oxygen	Yes: long-term oxygen from 5 months	Yes: long-term oxygen from 9 months
CPAP	–	Yes: 2 weeks during LRTI	–	–	–
BiPAP	–	–	From 29 months	–	–
Cardiac issues	–	Cardiomegaly	Pulmonary hypertension	Mitral regurgitation, patent foramen ovale and PDA	–
Feeding	NGT	NGT	NGT	NGT	PO
Surgery	Nil	Nil	Nil	Nil	Bilateral herniotomy: 4 months VP shunt insertion: 31 months
General anaesthetic	–	–	–	–	1st: standard intubation aged 4 months 2nd: NPA and LMA with catheter exchange to ETT. Tube found to be positional due to tracheomalacia, GlideScope used to reposition tube
Otological complications	–	–	EAC stenosis and recurrent otitis externa	–	–
Cause of death	Respiratory failure	Unknown	Respiratory failure	Respiratory failure and failed intubation	–

Ear disease was documented in one patient (patient 3). Soft tissue narrowing of the ear canals in this patient predisposed them to recurrent episodes of otitis externa. No documented cases of conductive hearing loss, sensorineural hearing loss, recurrent acute otitis media or chronic suppurative otitis media were found within the records, although this is likely to be an underestimation. Difficulty testing thresholds in these patients with cognitive impairment and multiple co-morbidities is likely to have influenced the information available in a retrospective study such as this. Certainly, ear disease is a clinical feature in several other lysosomal storage diseases, such as mucopolysaccharidosis (Simmons et al. 2005).

Teams Involved in Patient Care

Multidisciplinary working was vital for all patients with hospital-based input from neonatal, general, respiratory, cardiac and metabolic paediatricians, geneticists, ENT and general surgeons, speech and language therapists, dieticians and physiotherapists. A large part of each patient's management was community based with complex community teams required to enable them to be at home with nursing care, respite and hospice involvement.

Discussion

A comprehensive literature search revealed only eight articles linking I-cell disease to the specific ENT search terms (Table 1). Our patient cohort has revealed several important areas that highlight a need for an awareness of the ENT manifestations in patients with I-cell disease.

Airway Issues

Anaesthetic difficulties are well reported in the literature due to multiple factors. Mucopolysaccharide deposits have been reported in the airways of patients with I-cell disease leading to a grossly thickened epiglottis, larynx, trachea and tongue base (Peters et al. 1985). This occurs as a result of the lack of lysosomal enzymes which leads to macro-molecules in the lysosome causing an abnormal architecture (Hanai et al. 1971). This process complicates the airway of I-cell patients who already have other predisposing cranio-facial causes of upper airway obstruction. Such craniofacial issues combined with adenotonsillar hypertrophy result in obstructive sleep apnoea (OSA) being almost universal in these patients. Often the risks of an anaesthetic mean that surgical management is not feasible and as such medical management with continuous positive airway pressure (CPAP) is used.

In a recent case review of three patients, the problems encountered with managing their airways were reviewed. In all three cases, the patient required emergency intubation. Difficulties were encountered with simple face mask ventilation as well as with the use of supraglottic devices such as the laryngeal mask airway (LMA), attributed to the presence of significant 'deposits' in the upper airway distorting the normal anatomy. The authors highlighted that LMAs may offer a temporary solution but may not be successful in securing the airway. Direct laryngoscopy by the otolaryngology team enabled the airway to be secured in all three patients and was recommended as the best approach to intubation (Mallen et al. 2015).

Guidance has now been published with advice regarding safe intubation of I-cell patients (Roth et al. 2015). This guidance reinforces the difficulties that can be faced with even face mask ventilation and oral airway adjuncts. The recommendation is to have a full multidisciplinary experienced team and to ensure that a difficult airway algorithm is followed. Importantly a recent review (Hakim et al. 2017) has revealed that the status of a child's airway with I-cell disease deteriorates with age, so it is vital to be prepared to encounter difficulties even in the context of a patient that has previously had an uncomplicated anaesthetic. This has

been demonstrated within our patient cohort with our patient number 5 undergoing two anaesthetic procedures: the first being uncomplicated at age 4 months and the second resulting in reintubation and the use of a GlideScope at aged 31 months.

Patient 4 had a failed emergency intubation during an acute respiratory illness while at a non-specialist hospital. As a result of this event, certain recommendations have been made: firstly that in the event of severe respiratory distress, children with I-cell disease should where possible be transferred to a specialist centre as a matter of urgency and secondly that a regular 'airway plan' should be made with families to discuss and decide if intubation should be attempted both in an acute and an elective setting and how the child should be managed in a palliative way if not. If intubation is to be attempted during acute decompensations, then this should ideally be managed in a setting where the high risks can be minimalized.

Respiratory Issues

A number of pulmonary complications have been described including the mucosal thickening which can extend throughout the lower respiratory tract. Other findings include lipid granulomata (Gilbert et al. 1972), chronic respiratory infections, restrictive lung disease due a small thoracic cage, pulmonary haemorrhage and congestion and focal indurations due to bronchopneumonic infiltrations (Ishak et al. 2012).

Within our patient series, respiratory failure was evident throughout, but each patient had differing respiratory requirements. The use of supplemental oxygen for comfort and to maintain saturations over 92% was universal with prolonged assisted ventilatory support in only one case and interval CPAP in one patient during a lower respiratory tract infection.

Nasal CPAP has been found to be beneficial in overcoming the increased airway resistance caused by the anatomical deformities, increased secretions and recurrent atelectasis often associated with the frequent lower respiratory tract infections (LRTI) that are encountered in these patients. In a case report by Sheikh et al., they describe the use of CPAP leading to a significant reduction in morbidity by decreasing the impact of the patients OSA on their respiratory effort (Sheikh et al. 1998).

From our experience, we found that non-invasive ventilation was considered in patients that showed evidence of obstructed breathing or had a raised AHI, but if possible its use was avoided as given the prognosis; comfort was the overriding priority. One of our patients required BiPAP support 24 h a day. This is an unusual undertaking as normal practice is to not extend this beyond 16 h a day. In this particular patient, parents felt that the child was more comfortable with the NIV rather than without it, and it was felt that it enabled the family to have more time with the patient resulting in a better quality of life. From comparing age at death, it might also be the case that in doing so prolonged the patient's life with age at death being by far the greatest at 97 weeks. This highlights the patient-specific approach that needs to be taken with appropriate counselling of the implications of the treatments we impose or suggest.

Cardiac Issues

During respiratory tract infections, OSA symptoms can worsen with associated increased morbidity due to hypoxia, right heart strain, hypoventilation and eventually pulmonary hypertension and congestive heart failure. Congestive heart failure in I-cell patients is therefore often multifactorial with a contribution from underlying hypertrophic or dilated cardiomyopathy, aortic and mitral valve thickening (Eminoglu et al. 2016) as well as the OSA.

Gastroenterological Issues

After airway, respiratory and cardiac issues, the most common clinical problem is poor growth. It has been reported that from birth babies with I-cell should be able to safely coordinate an adequate suck reflex to be able to feed, but often they are not able to meet their nutritional requirements due to respiratory issues making feeding difficult resulting in nasogastric feeding tubes being placed (Leroy et al. 2012). Difficulty ensuring adequate oral nutrition is often progressive, reflecting worsening efficiency of swallow and aspiration risk, resulting from the distortion of oropharyngeal and laryngopharyngeal anatomy by disease 'deposits'. Therefore, affected children may have to be considered for long-term feeding support, with the decision necessitating careful consideration due to anaesthetic risks associated with gastrostomy tube insertion. This is seen within our case series with four of the patients requiring NGT feed supplementation of whom 100% were deemed unfit for elective surgery. While difficulty feeding is almost universal, care must be taken with enteral supplementation as a normal weight will not be desirable given the extreme short stature. Care must be taken to aim for an appropriate weight for length; assessment of the mid-upper arm circumference may also be a useful guide to appropriate nutritional intake.

Phenotypic Variations

Patient 2 died aged 4 months despite being diagnosed early at 2 weeks and had severe respiratory effects of the disease.

Their older sibling died aged 19 months despite it taking 2 months to achieve a diagnosis as she had less severe respiratory involvement. This leads to a conclusion that age of diagnosis is not necessarily related to disease survival. This is likely to be the case as much of the management of such patients involves best supportive care which can be offered in the absence of disease classification.

Conclusions

I-cell disease remains a severely life-limiting condition with management strategies focused upon maintaining quality of life and palliation.

Our patients have revealed two genetic variants with differing phenotypic features. Despite the differences, some common themes persist. Respiratory failure and airway problems including sleep-disordered breathing were ubiquitous in this cohort.

Any intervention requiring a general anaesthetic needs careful multidisciplinary consideration due to significant associated risks and possibly death. Management as a result is generally multidisciplinary, non-surgical and symptomatic.

This case series demonstrates universal involvement of the airway and respiratory systems, an important consideration when selecting meaningful outcomes for future effectiveness studies of novel therapies.

Acknowledgements   Not applicable.

Summary

Readers will gain an insight into the presenting features of I-cell disease with a detailed discussion of the airway and respiratory manifestations of the disease including a discussion over appropriate management approaches.

Declarations

Ethics Approval and Consent to Participate

Ethical approval was not needed.

Consent for Publication

Informed consent was obtained from all patients for which identifying information is included in this article.

Availability of Data and Material

All data generated or analysed during this study are included in the published article.

Completing Interests

Not applicable.

Funding

Not applicable.

Authors' Contributions

Edmiston, R. – Data collection, interpretation and primary author.

Wilkinson, S. – Data interpretation and draft review. Senior author respiratory section.

Jones, S. – Data interpretation and draft review. Senior author genetics section.

Tylee, K. – Data interpretation and genetic analysis

Broomfield, A. – Genetic analysis.

Bruce, I. A. – Data collection, interpretation and senior reviewing author.

All authors read and approved the final article.

References

Brouillette RT, Morielli A, Leimanis A, Waters KA, Luciano R, Ducharme FM (2000) Nocturnal pulse oximetry as an abbreviated testing modality for pediatric obstructive sleep apnea. Pediatrics 105:405–412

Cathy SS, Kudo M, Tiede S, Raas-Rothschild A, Braulke T, McKusick VA (2008) Molecular order in mucolipidosis II and III nomenclature. Am J Med Genet A 146(5):512–513

Eminoglu F, Yaman A, Kendrili T, Odek C, Ucar T (2016) Mucolipidosis type II (I-cell disease) with pulmonary hypertension and difficult airway. Mol Genet Metab 117(2):S45

Gilbert EF, Dawson G, zu Rhein GM, Opitz KM, Spranger JW (1972) I-cell disease, mucolipidosis II pathological, histochemical ultrastructural and biochemical observations in four cases. Z Kinderheilkd 114:259–292

Hakim M, Walia H, Krishna S, Tobias J (2017) Anaesthetic management of a 13 years old adolescent with mucolipidosis type II for total hip arthroplasty. J Med Cases 8(7):203–206

Hanai J, Leroy J, O'Brien JS (1971) Ultrastructure of cultured fibroblasts in I-cell disease. Am J Dis Child 122(1):34–38

Ishak M, Zambrano E, Bazzy-Asaad A, Esquibies A (2012) Unusual pulmonary findings in mucolipidosis II. Pediatr Pulmonol 47(7):719–721

Leroy G, Cathey S, Friez M (2012) Mucolipidosis II. Gene Reviews. http://www.ncbi.nlm.nih.gov/books/NBK1828/

Lynch SA, Crushell E, Lambert D, Bryne N et al (2018) Catalogue of inherited disorders found among the Irish Traveller population. J Med Genet 55(4):233–239

Mallen J, Highstein M, Smith L, Cheng J (2015) Airway management considerations in children with I-cell disease. Int J Pediatr Otorhinolaryngol 79(5):760–762

Mueller T, Honey N, Little L (1983) Mucolipidosis II and III: the genetic relationships between two disorders of lysosomal enzyme biosynthesis. J Clin Invest 72(3):1016–1023

Peters ME, Arya S, Langer LO, Gilbert EF, Carlson R, Adkins W (1985) Narrow trachea in mucopolysaccharidoses. Pediatr Radiol 15:225–228

Roth W, Jones S, Beauve B, Dearlove O (2015) Anaesthesia recommendations for patients suffering from: mucolipidosis II and III. Anasthesiol Intensivmed 56(9):636–641

Sheikh S, Madiraju K, Qazi Q, Rao M (1998) Improved morbidity with the use of nasal continuous positive airway pressure in i-cell disease. Pediatr Pulmonol 25:128–129

Simmons MA, Bruce IA, Penney S, Wraith E, Rothera MP (2005) Otorhinolaryngological manifestations of the mucopolysaccharidoses. Int J Paediatr Otorhinolaryngol 69(5):589–595

Walker R, Allen D, Rothera M (1997) A fibreoptic intubation technique for children with mucopolysaccharidoses using the laryngeal mask airway. Paediatr Anaesth 7:421–426

Wiesmann UN, Herschkowitz NN (1981) Mucolipidosis II and III: the clinical pictures and pathogenetic mechanisms. Persp Inherit Metab Dis 4:437–451

JIMD Reports
DOI 10.1007/8904_2018_134

RESEARCH REPORT

Oral Ganglioside Supplement Improves Growth and Development in Patients with Ganglioside GM3 Synthase Deficiency

Heng Wang · Valerie Sency · Paul McJarrow ·
Alicia Bright · Qianyang Huang · Karen Cechner ·
Julia Szekely · JoAnn Brace · Andi Wang ·
Danting Liu · Angela Rowan · Max Wiznitzer ·
Aimin Zhou · Baozhong Xin

Received: 14 February 2018 / Revised: 1 June 2018 / Accepted: 8 June 2018 / Published online: 13 September 2018
© Society for the Study of Inborn Errors of Metabolism (SSIEM) 2018

Abstract Ganglioside GM3 synthase is a key enzyme involved in the biosynthesis of gangliosides. GM3 synthase deficiency (GM3D) causes an absence of GM3 and all downstream biosynthetic derivatives. The affected individuals manifest with severe irritability, intractable seizures, and profound intellectual disability. The current study is to assess the effects of an oral ganglioside supplement to patients with GM3D, particularly on their growth and development during early childhood. A total of 13 young children, 11 of them under 40 months old, received oral ganglioside supplement through a dairy product enriched in gangliosides, for an average of 34 months. Clinical improvements were observed in most children soon after the supplement was initiated. Significantly improved growth and development were documented in these subjects as average percentiles for weight, height, and occipitofrontal circumference increased in 1–2 months. Three children with initial microcephaly demonstrated significant catch-up head growth and became normocephalic. We also illustrated brief improvements in developmental and cognitive scores, particularly in communication and socialization domains through Vineland-II. However, all improvements seemed transient and gradually phased out after 12 months of supplementation. Gangliosides GM1 and GM3, although measureable in plasma during the study, were not significantly changed with ganglioside supplementation for up to 30 months. We speculate that the downstream metabolism of ganglioside biosynthesis is fairly active and the potential need for gangliosides in the human body is likely substantial. As we search for new effective therapies for GM3D, approaches to reestablish endogenous ganglioside supplies in the affected individuals should be considered.

Communicated by: Roberto Giugliani, MD, PhD

Electronic supplementary material: The online version of this chapter (https://doi.org/10.1007/8904_2018_134) contains supplementary material, which is available to authorized users.

H. Wang · V. Sency · A. Bright · K. Cechner · J. Szekely · J. Brace · A. Wang · B. Xin
DDC Clinic - Center for Special Needs Children, Middlefield, OH, USA

H. Wang · M. Wiznitzer
Department of Pediatrics, Case Western Reserve University School of Medicine, Cleveland, OH, USA

H. Wang · M. Wiznitzer
Rainbow Babies & Children's Hospital, Cleveland, OH, USA

H. Wang (✉)
Department of Molecular Cardiology, Cleveland Clinic, Cleveland, OH, USA
e-mail: wang@ddcclinic.org

P. McJarrow · A. Rowan
Fonterra Research and Development Centre, Palmerston North, New Zealand

Q. Huang · D. Liu · A. Zhou
Department of Chemistry, Center for Gene Regulation in Health and Diseases, Cleveland State University, Cleveland, OH, USA

Introduction

Ganglioside GM3 synthase (also called lactosylceramide alpha-2,3 sialyltransferase) is the key enzyme involved in the initial stages of the biosynthesis of the a-, b-, c-series gangliosides. The enzyme deficiency (OMIM 609056) is a rare metabolic disorder inherited as an autosomal recessive trait, initially reported in the Old Order Amish

(Simpson et al. 2004), and later found in other ethnic groups as well (Boccuto et al. 2014; Fragaki et al. 2013). In patients with GM3 synthase deficiency (GM3D), GM3 and all downstream biosynthetic derivatives in the circulation are extremely low and scarcely detectable even with some recently improved analytic assays (Huang et al. 2014, 2016). Although the pathological mechanism remains to be understood, the condition is severe, characterized with infantile onset of severe irritability, failure to thrive, developmental stagnation, cortical blindness, profound intellectual disability, and intractable seizures (Boccuto et al. 2014; Farukhi et al. 2006; Fragaki et al. 2013; Simpson et al. 2004; Wang et al. 2013, 2016).

The treatment of the condition remains challenging. However, it has been noted that most children affected with the condition are clinically symptom-free for a period of time after birth, which implies that the infants might be protected in utero from the negative effects of ganglioside synthase deficiency. One possible explanation is that the maternal provision of gangliosides through the placenta during pregnancy might keep the newborns from developing clinical symptoms. The disease then progresses quickly after birth and causes significant constitutional impairments in growth and development by 6 months of age (Wang et al. 2016), as the maternal provision of gangliosides is terminated at birth and progressively depleted afterward. If this is the case, we might be able to relieve, partially relieve, or even prevent some symptoms by providing an adequate amount of gangliosides to affected children during the early stages of the disease, particularly before their symptoms develop. Based on this hypothesis, we designed this study to assess the effects of providing oral ganglioside supplement to patients with GM3D during infancy and early childhood with emphasis on their growth and development.

Materials and Methods

Patients and Experimental Design

The study (ClinicalTrials.gov Identifier: NCT02234024) was approved by the IRB of DDC Clinic, Center for Special Needs Children in Middlefield, Ohio, and written informed consent was obtained from patients' legal guardians. The study protocol (Supplementary Table 1) was presented to the parents of children diagnosed with GM3D and younger than 40 months. All study participants' diagnosis was confirmed with a homozygous mutation c.862C>T (p.R288*) in *ST3GAL5* gene identified through DNA sequencing as described previously (Wang et al. 2016). Fifteen of them chose to participate in the study and received oral ganglioside supplement. Two patients older than 40 months at the time also received oral ganglioside

supplement per parents' request, and they were included in the study with emphasis on the clinical aspect.

All study participants received Ganglioside 500™ (G500, Fonterra Co-operative Group Ltd), a commercial pediatric grade food product prepared from the milk fat globule membrane of bovine cream, manufactured to GMP standard, and tested and standardized during production. It contained relatively high levels of gangliosides (5 mg GM3 and 6 mg GD3/g of G500 powder) compared to milk and was administered at a starting dose of 0.5 g/kg body weight/day, divided evenly in a daily dietary regimen. The dosage was adjusted up to 2 g/kg body weight/day based on patients' tolerance, with 0.5 g/kg body weight/day as the minimal acceptable dosage to be included in the final data analysis, as it was the dosage we found effective in three individuals receiving ganglioside supplements from pork brain prior to this study. The duration of the supplementation to be included in the study was either more than 24 months or no less than 12 months with the supplement ongoing. Four patients were excluded from the study as they either took the supplement insufficiently or irregularly based on the parameters we set as described above.

The patients were evaluated at baseline, 1, 2, 4, and 6 months, and then every 3 months afterward for an additional 24 months with a total of 30 months or more according to the study protocol (Supplementary Table 1). The clinical evaluations for all individuals were performed by the same physician across the study. At each visit, growth and development were assessed; the parent questionnaire along with seizure and irritability log sheets recorded by families was reviewed; and blood samples were collected for ganglioside measurements.

Developmental and Other Assessments

Developmental and cognitive evaluations were performed through Vineland Adaptive Behavior Scales – Second Edition (Vineland-II) at the beginning of the study and every 6 months afterward for each subject by the same developmental specialist. The domains assessed through Vineland-II included communication, daily living skills, socialization, and motor skills.

Auditory evaluations with otoacoustic emissions (OAE) and auditory brainstem response (ABR) were performed at the beginning of the study and every 12 months afterward up to 24 months. Electroencephalogram (EEG) and brain MRI were selectively performed either as a part of the study or as clinically indicated.

Biochemical Assays

The blood samples were collected at each visit and kept at −80°C. Gangliosides including GM1, GM2, and GM3 were analyzed with a reverse-phase ultra-performance liquid chromatography (UPLC)/tandem mass spectrometry (MS) method as described recently (Huang et al. 2016).

Data Analysis and Statistics

As GM3D is an extremely rare metabolic disorder, the statistical methods applied were mainly descriptive. All data, expressed as numbers or percentiles, were presented as means ± SD.

Results

Clinical Observation

Eleven younger patients (8 females and 3 males), aged from birth to 39 months (14 ± 13 months) with 6 of them under 12 months old, along with 2 older patients aged 7.3 and 9.6 years, with GM3D received ganglioside supplements for an average of 34 (12–56) months, with 10 of 13 subjects still receiving the supplement, while the study was summarized (Table 1). No significant side effects were reported in these individuals during the time of ganglioside administration. The parents were given a choice after a 24-month trial; eight children continued the supplement, while three patients discontinued with various rationales

from parents including its inconvenience (No. 1), possible allergy to the product (No. 3), and pursuit of other treatment options (No. 6).

At the beginning of the study, all patients demonstrated various clinical manifestations, including failed hearing screening, severe irritability, hypotonia, failure to thrive, developmental delay, and seizures. Clinical responses were observed in 12 out of 13 patients by the physician and in 11 out of 13 patients by parents during the study (Table 1 and Supplementary Table 2), with improved eye contact in the younger patients and decreased irritability in the older patients being the most frequent and prominent findings by both parents and physician. Improved eye contact and increased responsiveness to the environment, while trivial, became more noticeable after 3–6 months of supplements, lasted approximately 12–24 months, and then slowly phased out.

Abnormal otoacoustic emissions (OAE) were observed in all subjects during the auditory evaluations before G500 supplement. Auditory brainstem response (ABR) was completed only in three children because of difficulties in assessment under minimal sedations. However, all three children demonstrated abnormal ABR findings. The abnormal OAE was normalized after 12-month supplementation of G500 in an infant who received G500 supplement soon after birth (No. 3) but remained abnormal in other children

Table 1 Clinical information of patients at the study

ID	Gender	Age at start (months)	G500 dosage (g/kg body/day)	Study duration (months)	Current status	Clinical responses observed by the clinician/parents and most prominent findings[a]
1	Female	31	1.0	30	Discontinued	+/+, improved eye contact and muscle strength
2	Female	14	2.0	30	Ongoing	+/−, improved eye contact and weight gain
3	Female	0	1.0	27	Discontinued	+/+, normalized hearing, improved eye contact. and decreased irritability
4	Male	13	1.0	56	Ongoing	+/+, increased interaction, more alert. and smiling
5	Female	39	1.5	56	Ongoing	+/+, decreased irritability which returned when she was off formula
6	Female	27	1.5	36	Discontinued	+/+, improved interaction
7	Male	5	0.7	26	Ongoing	+/+, improved eye contact and decreased irritability
8	Female	7	2.0	39	Ongoing	+/+, responded to visual stimuli and decreased constipation
9	Female	8	1.0	12	Ongoing	+/+, improved eye contact and object tracking
10	Female	6	2.0	47	Ongoing	+/+, improved eye contact, and good weight gain with a growth pattern similar to normal children
11	Male	2	2.0	20	Ongoing	−/−
12	Male	115	0.5	24	Ongoing	+/+, decreased irritability
13	Male	87	1.0	36	Ongoing	+/+, decreased irritability and increased interactions

[a] + and − represent positive and negative clinical responses observed by the clinician/parents, respectively

Table 2 Growth parameters and ganglioside levels in GM3D patients receiving G500

Time (months)	0	1	2	4	6	9	12	15	18	21	24	27	30
Weight percentile	6 ± 10 (2/11)	8 ± 14 (2/11)	7 ± 13 (2/11)	5 ± 11 (2/11)	4 ± 8 (2/11)	7 ± 15 (2/11)	6 ± 15 (2/11)	5 ± 11 (2/10)	6 ± 12 (2/10)	5 ± 9 (2/10)	2 ± 5 (2/10)	3 ± 6 (2/9)	3 ± 5 (2/8)
Height percentile	12 ± 10 (6/11)	15 ± 20 (6/11)	23 ± 33 (6/11)	16 ± 24 (6/11)	13 ± 30 (6/11)	16 ± 25 (5/11)	11 ± 26 (3/11)	10 ± 17 (3/10)	12 ± 14 (3/10)	7 ± 9 (3/10)	5 ± 12 (3/10)	9 ± 12 (3/9)	3 ± 4 (3/8)
OFC percentile	12 ± 26 (3/11)	14 ± 26 (4/11)	12 ± 23 (5/11)	11 ± 19 (5/11)	9 ± 15 (6/11)	5 ± 6 (5/11)	6 ± 7 (5/11)	6 ± 7 (4/10)	6 ± 7 (4/10)	6 ± 6 (4/10)	7 ± 10 (3/10)	7 ± 8 (3/9)	2 ± 2 (2/8)
GM1 (ng/mL)	924 ± 292	990 ± 157	1,035 ± 196	968 ± 319	829 ± 193	895 ± 192	952 ± 223	930 ± 257	838 ± 203	848 ± 275	1,047 ± 278	962 ± 293	738 ± 292
GM3 (ng/mL)	86 ± 26	84 ± 18	103 ± 23	95 ± 15	87 ± 15	89 ± 12	88 ± 20	103 ± 30	76 ± 15	85 ± 18	95 ± 33	83 ± 16	85 ± 21

Data are expressed as means ± SD with the numbers of children in the normal range (between 5th and 95th percentile) over the total amount of children participating in the study in the parentheses

in follow-up auditory studies. The series EEG and brain MRI performed before and during the G500 supplement showed no significant changes throughout the study.

Growth

Improved growth was observed soon after G500 supplement started in the majority of children participating in the study. A catch-up growth became noticeable in some individuals as soon as 1 month after the supplementation started, and as a result, the average percentiles for weight, height, and occipitofrontal circumference (OFC) were increased (Table 2). Three children manifesting with microcephaly (OFC less than the 5th percentile) at the beginning of the study demonstrated significant catch-up growth of the head after 1–6 months of the supplement, as the OFC in these children moved up to the normal range (Table 2). Several children demonstrated growth patterns completely different from the typical patterns of weight, height, and OFC that we observed in GM3D children without G500 supplement (Fig. 1). One female (No. 10) was able to maintain weight, height, and OFC in the normal range until 4.5 years old (Fig. 1g–i). This growth pattern was not observed in any affected children in previous natural history studies. However, we noted that these improvements did not last and slowly phased out after 12 months of supplements in most children. The growth pattern seemed to return to the typical growth pattern reported in the children with GM3D, even if they continued to receive the supplement.

Developmental and Cognitive Evaluation

Developmental and cognitive scores were substantially low in GM3D children at the beginning of the study, as demonstrated by lower scores in Vineland-II. Increasing raw scores were observed in all domains with the G500 supplement, with substantial jumps in scores after the first 6 months, followed by smaller but steady increases at each time point afterward. However, when the raw scores were standardized to domain standard scores with consideration of subjects' age, the improvements were only noticeable in socialization and communication domains soon after the supplementation started. No significant improvements were noted in daily living and motor skill domains. In fact, the standard scores generally declined in all domains over time of evaluation although the decline was less prominent in the socialization domain (Fig. 2 and Supplementary Table 3). It was also noted that patient 11 who had poor clinical response with the supplementation showed more substantially decreased domain scores.

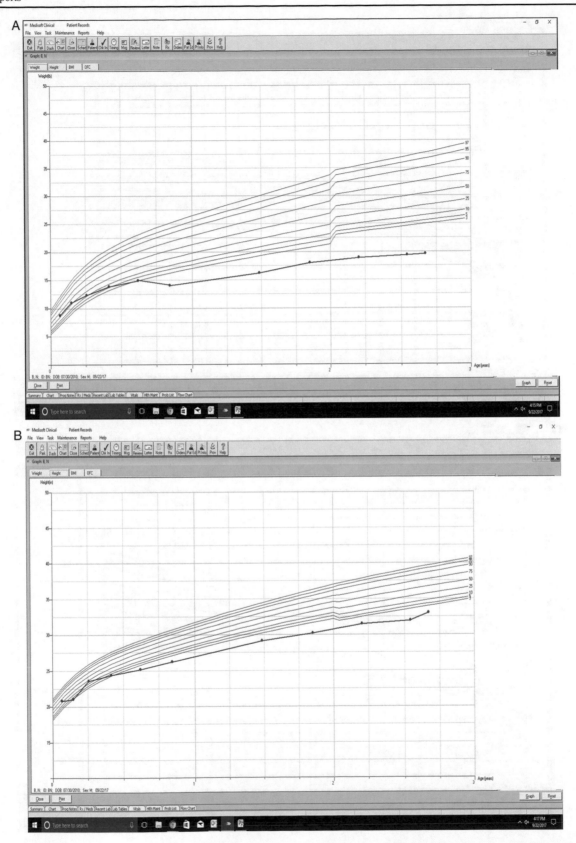

Fig. 1 Growth charts in GM3D patients. Growth charts for weight, height, and OFC are presented as (**a**), (**b**), and (**c**) for a patient who received no ganglioside supplement; (**d**), (**e**), and (**f**) for patient No. 4; and (**g**), (**h**), and (**i**) for patient No. 10, receiving G500 supplement at the age of 13 and 6 months, respectively, as indicated with red arrows

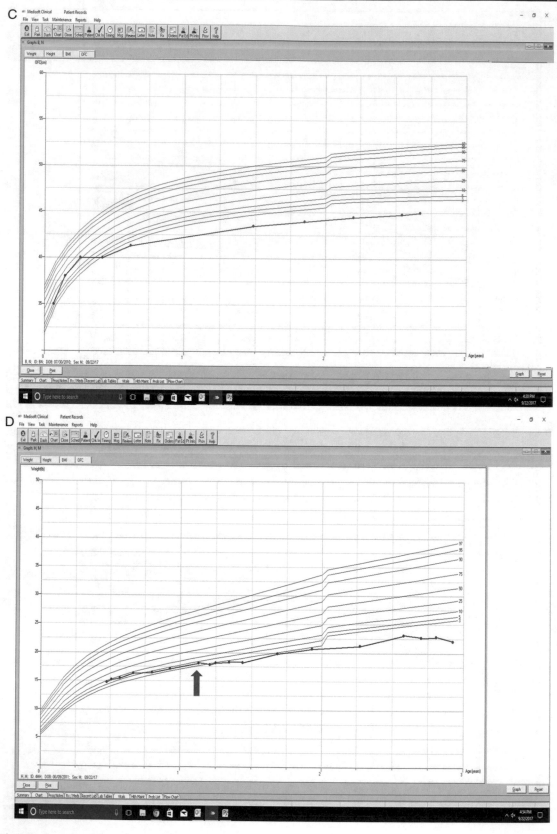

Fig. 1 (continued)

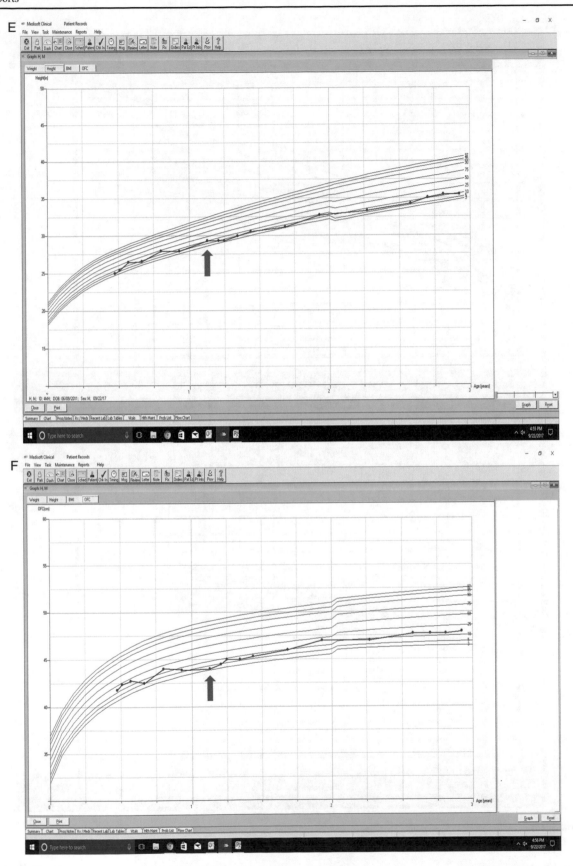

Fig. 1 (continued)

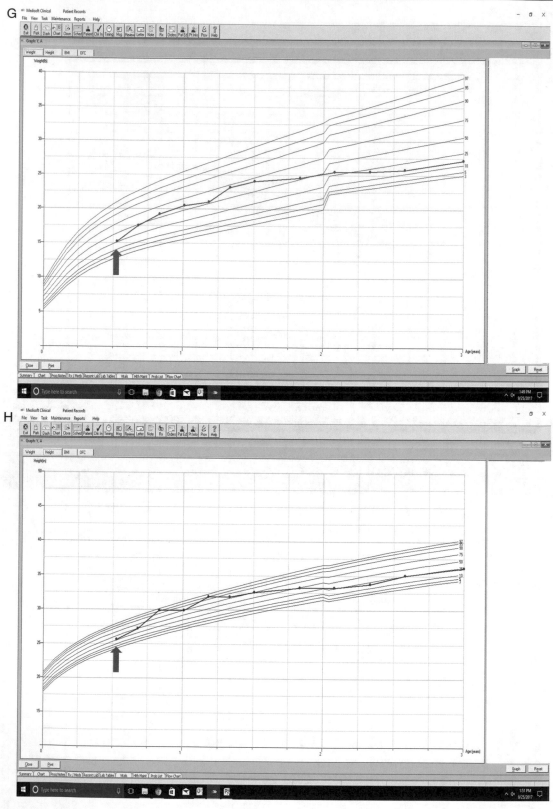

Fig. 1 (continued)

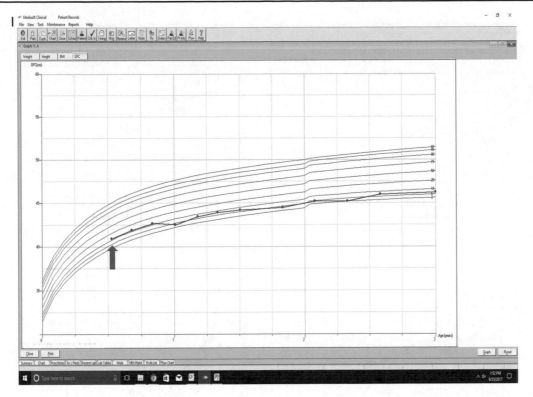

Fig. 1 (continued)

Plasma Ganglioside Levels

With the newly established UPLC/MS assay, GM3 was detected in all plasma samples from the patients with GM3D, although its abundance was only about 1% of the level observed in unaffected individuals (Huang et al. 2016). GM1 and GM3 were both measureable in all the plasma samples collected during the study, but no significant change was found in the levels of GM1 and GM3 before and after the G500 supplement was administered, for up to 30 months (Table 2). Plasma ganglioside GM2 was detectable only in a few random samples, and thus analyses are not presented here.

Discussion

Gangliosides as a group of multifunctional molecules are found on the surface of essentially all mammalian cells, particularly abundant in the central nervous system, where they represent about 10% of total lipid content. These sialic acid-containing glycosphingolipids are thought to function in the regulation of signaling pathways that impact cell proliferation, survival, adhesion, and motility, and they play essential roles in normal neural development and function (Schengrund 2015).

Genetic defects in the ganglioside biosynthesis pathway are devastating. Since we first reported a homozygous loss-of-function mutation c.862C>T (p.R288*) in *ST3GAL5* gene as the cause of GM3D in a group of Old Order Amish patients in 2004 (Simpson et al. 2004), more than 70 additional patients have been diagnosed, with some patients identified outside of the Amish community (Boccuto et al. 2014; Fragaki et al. 2013), indicating that this rare condition might be widespread. Several other genetic disorders along the ganglioside biosynthesis pathway have been reported recently, including mutations of the *B4GALNT1* (GM2 synthase) gene resulting in hereditary spastic paraplegia and cognitive impairment (Boukhris et al. 2013) and mutations in the *ST3GAL3* gene resulting in intellectual disability and West syndrome (Edvardson et al. 2013), all with severe consequences. These reports once again illustrate the critical roles that gangliosides play in human nervous system function and the need to find effective treatments for these conditions. The unique setting of our facility in providing medical care for most patients suffering from GM3D gives us an exceptional opportunity for such a study.

The exact pathological mechanism of this condition remains unclear as the metabolic consequences of the deficiency of GM3 synthase are manifold, including the lack of GM3 and its derivatives and the accumulation of lactosylceramide and its alternative metabolites. Mitochondrial dysfunction might also be involved as a part of the pathology since the significant decrease in mitochondrial

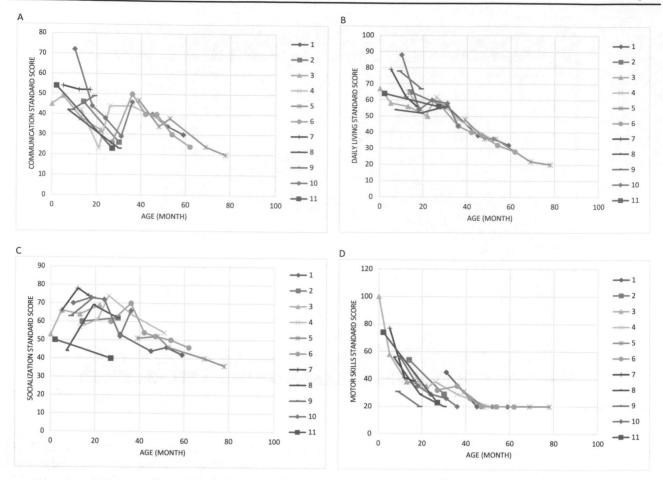

Fig. 2 Vineland-II domain scores in 11 GM3D patients receiving G500 during the study. (**a**) Communication domain, (**b**) daily living domain, (**c**) socialization domain, and (**d**) motor skill domain

membrane potential and increase in apoptosis were illustrated in the patients' fibroblasts (Fragaki et al. 2013). Several studies through gene-engineered animals have also provided important insights in understanding this condition and several other ganglioside metabolic disorders (Ohmi et al. 2014; Yoo et al. 2015; Yoshikawa et al. 2015).

By providing a significant amount of gangliosides orally during the early stages of the disease, this pilot study is the first clinical trial in seeking potential treatment for children with GM3D. The study is based on the hypothesis that maternal gangliosides coming across the placenta (Mitchell et al. 2012) overcome the inability of the affected fetus to synthesize gangliosides in the uterus and the oral supplement provided during very early childhood takes on the role maternal gangliosides play during pregnancy. Indeed, as a part of the natural history study, our earlier work has revealed that the children with GM3D had relatively normal intrauterine growth and development and showed minimal clinical symptoms at birth (Wang et al. 2013, 2016). Our previous study has also demonstrated that the amount of gangliosides in breast milk, although significantly higher

than infant formula, is not sufficient in maintaining normal growth and development or altering the disease course in the affected children as we found similar postnatal growth and developmental impairments in the children with GM3D regardless of whether they were breastfed or formula-fed (Wang et al. 2016). In this current study, through oral ganglioside supplementation, we have observed significant improvements in growth and development in the children with GM3D. This was not only reflected by reports from parents and clinical observations from physicians and other health professionals but also by improved growth parameters such as increased weight, height, and OFC when we compared them with the typical growth curves we described through our natural history study (Wang et al. 2016), along with improved developmental and cognitive scores, although the changes we identified were transient and slowly phased out.

It is noted that the abnormal hearing test identified in one newborn was normalized after 12-month supplementation and three children with microcephaly showed significant catch-up head growth and became normocephalic after

1–6-month supplementation (Table 2). These findings not only provide strong evidence supporting the efficacy of the oral dairy ganglioside supplementation but also give us hints that the pathology of this condition is potentially reversible. However, it is also noted that the responses to oral ganglioside supplements appeared more prominent in young infants than older children as many responses that we observed in younger children, such as the normalized hearing in a newborn and renormalized OFC in three infants, were not found in the older children. These findings suggest the importance of early intervention.

It is interesting to notice that the ganglioside levels in the plasma were not significantly changed after daily ganglioside supplementation for up to 30 months, although we observed noteworthy improved clinical symptoms, growth parameters, and developmental scores. It might be suspected that the gangliosides provided through oral supplements are not absorbed and utilized by these children as the ganglioside levels in the plasma were not significantly changed. However, earlier studies have documented that the gangliosides seemed readily absorbed and integrated into tissues as a higher content of gangliosides was found in the brain tissue of the breastfed infants compared with the formula-fed (Wang et al. 2003) and human breast milk contains significantly more GM3 compared with cow's milk and infant formulas (Pan and Izumi 2000). A more recent study further demonstrated that the supplementation of infant formula with gangliosides appeared to increase serum ganglioside levels in normal healthy infants (Gurnida et al. 2012). One may speculate that the downstream metabolism of ganglioside biosynthesis pathway is likely very active and the gangliosides absorbed in the circulation in these children have been taken up and metabolized by other organs and systems immediately; thus, no significant changes in serum ganglioside levels are observed. Indeed, GM3 synthase is a key enzyme involved in the initial stages of biosynthesis with multiple downstream pathways to various a-, b-, c-series gangliosides (Proia 2004), and the improvements of clinical symptoms, growth parameters, and developmental and cognitive scores appear with no significant changes on the serum gangliosides observed in children receiving oral supplementation. We are currently developing a new assay to determine if there are any changes for the gangliosides in the cellular components in these patients throughout the study. Further work through a stable isotope-labeled study in patients or through tissue ganglioside profile in animal studies would also be helpful in understanding this process.

The hypothesis that the amount of gangliosides needed in a human body is potentially substantial is also supported by other evidence. During the study, we found that GM3 and the downstream products in plasma samples collected from the umbilical cord of the genotypically positive newborn were detectable with the newly established sensitive method (Huang et al. 2016), but the levels are very similar to the levels we found in the older children (data not shown). These observations suggested that the plausibly massive needs of gangliosides during pregnancy and the maternal gangliosides transferred through the placenta to the fetus with the genetic defect may not be sufficient to meet their growth and development in the uterus. Indeed, the fact that most children with GM3D failed newborn hearing screening further supports this hypothesis as these infants might not receive enough maternal GM3 and the infants might be already affected at birth. It has been noted that maternal supplementation with a complex milk lipid mixture during pregnancy and lactation in rats can significantly increase the ganglioside contents in neonatal brain (Gustavsson et al. 2010); thus, the timeline of an early intervention might need to be redefined, considering as early as pregnancy.

In this study, we have observed some significant improvements in clinical symptoms, growth parameters, and developmental and cognitive scores through oral ganglioside supplement to the affected children. However, it remains concerning as the improvements we observed in this study are transient and slowly phase out during the study. As we further explore therapeutic options for GM3D, such as supplemental studies with considerably larger amounts of gangliosides than the amounts we used in this study or given through parenteral pathways, we should also consider the approaches to reestablish endogenous ganglioside supplies with abundance such as hematopoietic stem cell or liver transplantation and gene therapies in the affected individuals. An additional critical factor to be considered to warrant the ultimate effective outcome is an adequate amount of gangliosides in the maternal blood during pregnancy.

Acknowledgments We thank the families for their patience and support. We appreciate many physicians who provided outstanding and compassionate care to the children affected by the disease. The study was supported in part by Fonterra (via the New Zealand Primary Growth Partnership program, funded by Fonterra Co-operative Group Ltd and the NZ Ministry for Primary Industries) and the Zverina Family Foundation.

One Sentence Take-Home Message

Oral ganglioside supplement significantly improves growth and development in patients with ganglioside GM3 synthase deficiency; however, the improvements seem transient and gradually phase out after 12 months.

Contributions of Individual Authors

All authors participated in the conduct of the study, and Heng Wang, Paul McJarrow, Aimin Zhou, and Baozhong Xin contributed to the planning and reporting of the work.

The Authors Who Serves as Guarantor

Heng Wang

Competing Interest

Heng Wang, as a principal investigator, received funding support from Fonterra Co-operative Group Ltd. to DDC Clinic for this study and also served as a speaker for a Fonterra-organized symposium. Paul McJarrow and Angela Rowan are employees of Fonterra.

Funding

The study was supported in part by Fonterra (via the New Zealand Primary Growth Partnership program, funded by Fonterra Co-operative Group Ltd and the NZ Ministry for Primary Industries) and Zverina Family Foundation. The authors confirm independence from the sponsors; the content of the article has not been influenced by the sponsors.

Ethics Approval and Patients Consent

The study was approved by the DDC Clinic IRB, and written informed consent was obtained from the patients' legal guardians and available upon request (ClinicalTrials.gov Identifier: NCT02234024).

References

Boccuto L, Aoki K, Flanagan-Steet H, Chen CF et al (2014) A mutation in a ganglioside biosynthetic enzyme, ST3GAL5, results in salt & pepper syndrome, a neurocutaneous disorder with altered glycolipid and glycoprotein glycosylation. Hum Mol Genet 23:418–433

Boukhris A, Schule R, Loureiro JL et al (2013) Alteration of ganglioside biosynthesis responsible for complex hereditary spastic paraplegia. Am J Hum Genet 93:118–123

Edvardson S, Baumann AM, Mühlenhoff M et al (2013) West syndrome caused by ST3Gal-III deficiency. Epilepsia 54: e24–e27

Farukhi F, Dakkouri C, Wang H et al (2006) Etiology of vision loss in ganglioside GM3 synthase deficiency. Ophthalmic Genet 27:89–91

Fragaki K, Ait-El-Mkadem S, Chaussenot A et al (2013) Refractory epilepsy and mitochondrial dysfunction due to GM3 synthase deficiency. Eur J Hum Genet 21:528–534

Gurnida DA, Rowan AM, Idjradinata P et al (2012) Association of complex lipids containing gangliosides with cognitive development of 6-month-old infants. Early Hum Dev 88:595–601

Gustavsson M, Hodgkinson SC, Fong B et al (2010) Maternal supplementation with a complex milk lipid mixture during pregnancy and lactation alters neonatal brain lipid composition but lacks effect on cognitive function in rats. Nutr Res 30:279–289

Huang Q, Zhou X, Liu D et al (2014) A new liquid chromatography/tandem mass spectrometry method for quantification of gangliosides in human plasma. Anal Biochem 455:26–34

Huang Q, Liu D, Xin B et al (2016) Quantification of monosialogangliosides in human plasma through chemical derivatization for signal enhancement in LCeESI-MS. Anal Chim Acta 929:31–38

Mitchell MD, Henare K, Balakrishnan B et al (2012) Transfer of gangliosides across the human placenta. Placenta 33:312–316

Ohmi Y, Ohkawa Y, Tajima O et al (2014) Ganglioside deficiency causes inflammation and neurodegeneration via the activation of complement system in the spinal cord. J Neuroinflammation 11:61

Pan XL, Izumi T (2000) Variation of the ganglioside compositions of human milk, cow's milk and infant formulas. Early Hum Dev 57:25–31

Proia RL (2004) Gangliosides help stabilize the brain. Nat Genet 36:1147–1148

Schengrund CL (2015) Gangliosides: glycosphingolipids essential for normal neural development and function. Trends Biochem Sci 40:397–406

Simpson MA, Cross H, Proukakis C et al (2004) Infantile-onset symptomatic epilepsy syndrome caused by a homozygous loss-of-function mutation of GM3 synthase. Nat Genet 36:1225–1229

Wang B, McVeagh P, Petocz P et al (2003) Brain ganglioside and glycoprotein sialic acid in breastfed compared with formula-fed infants. Am J Clin Nutr 78:1024–1029

Wang H, Bright A, Xin B et al (2013) Cutaneous dyspigmentation in patients with ganglioside GM3 synthase deficiency. Am J Med Genet 161A:875–879

Wang H, Wang A, Wang D et al (2016) Early growth and development impairment in patients with ganglioside GM3 synthase deficiency. Clin Genet 89:625–629

Yoo SW, Motari MG, Susuki K et al (2015) Sialylation regulates brain structure and function. FASEB J 29:3040–3053

Yoshikawa M, Go S, Suzuki SI et al (2015) Ganglioside GM3 is essential for the structural integrity and function of cochlear hair cells. Hum Mol Genet 24:2796–2807

JIMD Reports
DOI 10.1007/8904_2018_131

RESEARCH REPORT

Feeding Difficulties and Orofacial Myofunctional Disorder in Patients with Hepatic Glycogen Storage Diseases

Chenia Caldeira Martinez · Tássia Tonon ·
Tatiéle Nalin · Lilia Farret Refosco ·
Carolina Fischinger Moura de Souza ·
Ida Vanessa Doederlein Schwartz

Received: 29 January 2018 / Revised: 26 June 2018 / Accepted: 27 July 2018 / Published online: 22 September 2018
© Society for the Study of Inborn Errors of Metabolism (SSIEM) 2018

Abstract Hepatic glycogen storage diseases (GSDs) are inborn errors of metabolism whose dietary treatment involves uncooked cornstarch administration and restriction of simple carbohydrate intake. The prevalence of feeding difficulties (FDs) and orofacial myofunctional disorders (OMDs) in these patients is unknown. *Objective*: To ascertain the prevalence of FDs and OMDs in GSD. *Methods*: This was a cross-sectional, prospective study of 36 patients (19 males; median age, 12.0 years; range, 8.0–18.7 years) with confirmed diagnoses of GSD (type Ia = 22; Ib = 8; III = 2; IXa = 3; IXc = 1). All patients were being treated by medical geneticists and dietitians. Evaluation included a questionnaire for evaluation of feeding behavior, the orofacial myofunctional evaluation (AMIOFE), olfactory and taste performance (Sniffin' Sticks and Taste Strips tests), and facial anthropometry. *Results*: Nine (25%) patients had decreased olfactory perception, and four (11%) had decreased taste perception for all flavours. Eight patients (22.2%) had decreased perception for sour taste. Twenty-six patients (72.2%) had FD, and 18 (50%) had OMD. OMD was significantly associated with FD, tube feeding, selective intake, preference for fluid and semisolid foods, and mealtime stress ($p < 0.05$). Thirteen patients (36.1%) exhibited mouth or oronasal breathing, which was significantly associated with selective intake ($p = 0.011$) and not eating together with the rest of the family ($p = 0.041$). Lower swallowing and chewing scores were associated with FD and with specific issues related to eating behavior ($p < 0.05$). *Conclusion*: There is a high prevalence of FDs and OMDs in patients with GSD. Eating behavior, decreased taste and smell perception, and orofacial myofunctional issues are associated with GSD.

Communicated by: Gerard T. Berry, M.D.

Electronic supplementary material: The online version of this chapter (https://doi.org/10.1007/8904_2018_131) contains supplementary material, which is available to authorized users.

C. C. Martinez (✉) · T. Tonon · T. Nalin · I. V. D. Schwartz
Post-graduate Program in Medicine: Medical Sciences, Universidade Federal do Rio Grande do Sul, Porto Alegre, Brazil
e-mail: chenia.martinez@gmail.com

L. F. Refosco · C. F. M. de Souza · I. V. D. Schwartz
Medical Genetics Service, Hospital de Clínicas de Porto Alegre, Porto Alegre, Brazil

I. V. D. Schwartz
Department of Genetics, Universidade Federal do Rio Grande do Sul, Porto Alegre, Brazil

Introduction

Hepatic glycogen storage diseases (GSDs) are inborn errors of glycogen metabolism. These conditions are divided into subtypes, depending on the enzyme defect involved (Wolfsdorf and Weinstein 2003; Walter et al. 2016). Phenotype depends on the disease subtype and extent of metabolic control, but major features include growth retardation, short stature, a doll-like face, hepatomegaly, hypoglycemia, hyperlactatemia, hypercholesterolemia, and hypertriglyceridemia (Chen and Kishnani 2012; Kishnani et al. 2014; Derks and Smit 2015).

Treatment can include restricted intake of simple carbohydrates (fructose, maltose, glucose, lactose, galactose), administration of uncooked cornstarch several times a day (including overnight, as some patients do not tolerate fasting for more than 3 h), and management of clinical and laboratory parameters (Weinstein and Wolfsdorf 2002; Chen and Kishnani 2012; Derks and Smit 2015). Sometimes, due to the dietary restrictions and continuous feeding

Springer

required, tube feeding is indicated to maintain normoglycemia and proper metabolic control (Rake et al. 2002; Weinstein and Wolfsdorf 2002; Flanagan et al. 2015).

Feeding difficulties (FDs) are common in childhood, affecting up to 50% of children regardless of sex or socioeconomic status. Causes include a variety of organic and behavioral issues, as well as the feeding style of the caregivers; specific features and severity vary widely (Carruth et al. 2004; Wright et al. 2007; Dunitz-Scheer et al. 2009; Mascola et al. 2010; Benjasuwantep et al. 2013; Edwards et al. 2015; Kerzner et al. 2015).

The main organic conditions associated with FDs are dysphagia; gastrointestinal, metabolic, and cardiorespiratory abnormalities; structural/mechanical abnormalities; orofacial myofunctional disorders (OMDs); growth failure; and tube feeding. Other issues that are also directly related include prolonged mealtimes, food refusal, mealtime stress, lack of autonomy to self-feed, lack of distractions to increase intake, difficulty in eating foods with different textures, and picky eating. FDs can cause significant nutritional and emotional problems in children and in their caregivers (Carruth et al. 2004; Wright et al. 2007; Dunitz-Scheer et al. 2009; Mascola et al. 2010; Benjasuwantep et al. 2013; Edwards et al. 2015; Kerzner et al. 2015).

Few studies have assessed the issue of OMD and FDs in patients with GSDs. This population is particularly susceptible to FDs, as both the disease and its treatment are associated with risk factors for the development of feeding disorders. Poor acceptance of dietary plans by patients and families is also a concern (Correia et al. 2008; Santos et al. 2014; Flanagan et al. 2015). Within this context, the present study aimed to investigate FDs, OMDs, and olfactory and gustatory perception in Brazilian patients with hepatic GSDs.

Materials and Methods

Sample

This was a cross-sectional, prospective study of 36 patients (19 males; median age, 12.0 years; range, 8.0–18.7 years) with confirmed diagnoses of GSD (type Ia, $n = 22$; Ib, $n = 8$; III, $n = 2$; IXa, $n = 3$; IXc, $n = 1$) who were being treated at Hospital de Clínicas de Porto Alegre, a referral center in Southern Brazil. Fifteen patients (41.7%) were being tube-fed, 12 (36.1%) through a gastrostomy. Three patients (8.3%) were on tube feeding due to severe food refusal, and five (13.8%) were fed either orally or by tube. Data were collected from 2015 to 2017. A convenience sampling strategy was used.

Due to similarities in clinical characteristics and treatment, GSD subtypes were pooled as "subtype I" (Ia and Ib)

and "other subtypes" (III and IX). Treatment included follow-up by an interdisciplinary team (a medical geneticist specializing in inborn errors of metabolism, a specialized dietitian, nurse, and clinical psychologist), with visits every 3 months; control of clinical and laboratory parameters; dietary management; and group therapy. Individuals under the age of 5 were excluded by recommendation of the tests. The study was approved by the Institutional Review Board of the hospital where it was carried out (protocol no. 150072), and written informed consent was obtained from all individuals before participation.

Procedures

Clinical information was collected from medical records and through a structured interview with the patient about FDs. To investigate dietary habits and feeding difficulties, a questionnaire of relevant items was constructed according to Edwards et al. (2015) and Kerzner et al. (2015); caregivers answered the questionnaire when patients were unable to understand the questions. Relevant behavioral signs and issues included selective intake, fear/aversion of feeding, prolonged mealtimes, mealtime stress (e.g., parents' and/or caregivers' insistence on offering food, constant resistance and/or refusal to feed, especially in childhood), preference for fluid/semisolid foods, and family eating habits (e.g., not eating together). Subjects were classified as having a "feeding difficulty" on the basis of the following three aspects: (1) self-report by patients/caregivers, (2) clinical evaluation by the researcher, and (3) presence of one or more of the aforementioned behaviors.

Clinical evaluations were performed on the same day by a trained speech–language pathologist with experience in administration of the study instruments, namely, (a) a validated protocol for investigation of OMD, the orofacial myofunctional evaluation with scores (AMIOFE) (De Felício and Ferreira 2008); (b) analysis of olfactory perception by the *Sniffin' Sticks* test (Hummel et al. 1997); and (c) Analysis of taste perception by the *Taste Strips* test (Mueller et al. 2003). This test evaluates four tastes (sweet, sour, salty, bitter), being possible to obtain the total score or the score of each flavor separately. For the present study, it were analyzed the total score and the sour taste, since sour taste is often present in foods restricted in the diet of patients with GSDs.

Statistical Analysis

The chi-square, Fisher's exact, Mann–Whitney U, and Spearman correlation tests were used for nonparametric variables, and Poisson regression with robust variance to analyze risk factors by prevalence ratio (PR). The

Kolmogorov–Smirnov test was used to evaluate the assumption of normality. The significance level was set at 5% ($p \leq 0.05$).

Results

Assessment of smell and taste perception was performed in 22 patients (61.1% of the sample), all aged ≥11 years, in accordance with the test recommendations. Regarding olfactory perception, the median score was 10.0 (8.8–11.2) points. Nine patients (40.9%) had median scores below the cutoff point, indicating hyposmia. For taste perception, the median score was 11.5 (10.0–14.0) points. Four patients (18.2%) had scores below the cutoff point for all flavors, suggesting hypogeusia. The scale for sourness alone ranges from 0 to 4 points. The sample median was 3.0 (0.8–3.0) points, with eight patients (36.4%) having a score indicative of decreased sour taste perception.

Variables related to the reduction of olfactory, gustatory, and sourness perception were compared to behavioral issues regarding food. Decreased olfactory perception was associated with selective intake ($p = 0.027$), while decreased sourness perception was associated with preference for fluid and/or semisolid foods ($p = 0.006$).

The prevalence of feeding issues (feeding behaviors or conditions that may impact on the child's feeding) and a comparison with the presence of FD are presented in Table 1. The overall prevalence of FD in this sample was 72.2% ($n = 26$). Since GSD I requires a more restrictive diet than other subtypes, the potential association between this subtype and FD needs to be investigated. In this study, we could not conduct a statistical comparison due to the discrepancy in sample size (30 participants with GSD I vs. 6 patients with other GSDs).

Findings related to feeding behavior were analyzed and compared to median scores in the orofacial myofunctional scale, specifically total, deglutition, and mastication scores (Table 2). The total orofacial myofunctional score correlated positively with age ($r = 0.493$, $p = 0.002$), suggesting that younger individuals had lower test scores.

Variables were analyzed by Poisson regression with robust variances to investigate risk factors for OMD, using prevalence ratios controlled by age. Preference for fluid/semisolid foods (PR = 10.29, 95% CI 1.4–75.1, $p = 0.021$) and selective intake (PR = 7.94, 95% CI 1.1–56.6, $p = 0.038$) were significant. This suggests that, even after controlling for age, these feeding issues are risk factors for OMD.

Table 3 presents an analysis of posture/appearance, mobility of orofacial structures, and orofacial functioning, stratified by age range (Table 3). Regarding stomatognathic functions, 1 patient presented with mouth breathing and 12 (33.33%) with oronasal-type breathing. Both breathing patterns were associated with selective intake ($p = 0.011$) and nonparticipation in family meals ($p = 0.014$). Mastication could not be assessed in three children due to lack of oral feeding secondary to complete food refusal. In these cases, the minimum score of one point was assigned, in accordance with test recommendations.

Table 1 Hepatic glycogen storage disorders: feeding aspects and feeding difficulty

	Sample prevalence ($n = 36$)	Feeding difficulty[a]		
	n (%)	Presence of feeding difficulty ($n = 26$)	Absence of feeding difficulty ($n = 10$)	*p-value
Tube feeding >1 year	15 (41.7%)	13 (50.0%)	2 (20.0%)	0.142
Exclusive breastfeeding <6 months	25 (69.4%)	21 (80.8%)	4 (40.0%)	0.039*
Feeding behaviors and conditions				
Selective intake	23 (63.9%)	22 (84.6%)	1 (10.0%)	<0.001*
Fear of feeding (or food aversion)	11 (30.6%)	11 (42.3%)	0 (0.0%)	0.016*
Preference for fluid/semisolid foods	21 (58.3%)	19 (73.1%)	2 (20.0%)	0.007*
Prolonged mealtimes	18 (50.0%)	14 (53.8%)	4 (40.0%)	0.360
Not eating together with the family	14 (38.8%)	14 (100%)	0 (0.0%)	0.003*
Mealtime stress	19 (52.8%)	16 (61.5%)	3 (30.0%)	0.139
Gastrointestinal conditions	13 (36.1%)	12 (46.2%)	1 (10.0%)	0.060

*Statistical significance by Fisher's Exact test to "feeding difficulty" ($p \leq 0.05$). Data presented by frequency (percentage)

[a] "Feeding difficulties" were determined on the basis of tree of these aspects: (1) self-reports by patients/family members, (2) clinical evaluation by the researcher, and (3) presence of one or more of the aforementioned behaviors

Table 2 Hepatic glycogen storage disorders: comparison between orofacial myofunctional evaluation scores with feeding aspects ($n = 36$)

	Scores of orofacial myofunctional evaluation					
	Total score	p-valor	Deglutition score	p-valor	Mastication score	p-valor
Tube feeding >1 year	84.0 (76.0–88.0)	0.012*	11.0 (9.0–13.0)	0.008*	5.0 (2.0–6.9)	0.077
Exclusive breastfeeding ≥6 months	87.0 (82.0–91.5)	0.256	12.0 (11.0–14.0)	0.728	5.0 (3.5–7.0)	0.446
Feeding difficulty	84.5 (81.2–90.0)	0.001*	12.0 (10.5–13.0)	0.001*	4.5 (3.0–6.0)	0.009*
Selective intake	84.0 (79.0–89.0)	<0.001*	12.0 (9.0–13.0)	0.004*	4.0 (2.0–6.0)	0.001*
Fear of feeding (or food aversion)	83.0 (69.0–90.0)	0.010*	11.0 (8.0–12.0)	0.015*	5.0 (1.0–6.0)	0.282
Preference for fluid/semisolid foods	84.0 (77.5–87.0)	<0.001*	11.0 (8.5–13.0)	<0.001*	5.0 (3.0–6.0)	0.051*
Prolonged mealtimes	84.0 (80.5–90.2)	0.038*	12.5 (11.0–14.0)	0.532	5.0 (2.7–7.0)	0.322
Not eating together with the family	84.6 (76.5–89.2)	0.019*	12.0 (8.0–12.2)	0.008*	5.0 (1.7–6.0)	0.088*
Mealtime stress	84.0 (79.0–90.0)	0.010*	12.0 (9.0–13.0)	0.058*	5.0 (3.0–6.0)	0.030*
Gastrointestinal conditions	85.0 (84.0–98.2)	0.339	12.0 (8.5–13.5)	0.152	5.0 (4.0–6.5)	0.690

*Statistical significance by Mann–Whitney test to "scores of orofacial myofunctional evaluation" ($p \leq 0.05$). Data presented by median (interquartile range)

Table 3 Hepatic glycogen storage disorders: children and adults in the specific abilities of orofacial myofunctional test

		Data by age range	
		Child ≤12 years old ($n = 22$)	Teenagers and adults >12 years old ($n = 14$)
	Reference score	Median (IQR)	Median (IQR)
Lips		3.0 (2.0–3.0)	3.0 (3.0–3.0)
Mandible/maxilla	3	2.0 (2.0–3.0)	3.0 (2.0–3.0)
Cheeks	3	2.0 (2.0–3.0)	3.0 (2.0–3.0)
Face	3	2.0 (2.0–3.0)	2.5 (2.0–3.0)
Tongue	3	3.0 (2.0–3.0)	3.0 (2.0–3.0)
Palate	3	3.0 (2.0–3.0)	3.0 (2.8–3.0)
Movements			
Lips	12	10.0 (9.8–11.3)	11.0 (9.5–12.0)
Tongue	18	17.0 (15.8–18.0)	18.0 (16.8–18.0)
Jaw	15	14.0 (12.0–15.0)	15.0 (14.8–15.0)
Cheeks	12	12.0 (10.8–12.0)	12.0 (11.0–12.0)
Functions			
Breathing	3	2.0 (2.0–3.0)	3.0 (3.0–3.0)
Deglutition	15	12.0 (11.0–13.0)	14.5 (11.8–15.0)
Mastication	10	5.0 (2.8–6.3)	7.0 (4.0–7.0)
Total	≥88	85.0 (81.3–90.3)	91.5 (84.8–99.0)

Data presented by median (IQR interquartile range)

Discussion

This was the first study in the literature to include a speech–language pathology viewpoint in the investigation of orofacial myofunctional issues and feeding behavior, as well as evaluate the possible association of these issues with the senses of smell and taste, in a sample of patients with hepatic glycogen storage diseases. Our findings indicate that feeding difficulties and orofacial myofunctional disorders are prevalent in this population, which may be particularly susceptible to the development of stomatognathic abnormalities.

GSD Ia was the most prevalent subtype in our sample, which is consistent with the literature (Janecke et al. 2001; Chou et al. 2002). Alternative feeding routes were used in a substantial portion of patients, which is consistent with the need for uninterrupted dietary treatment to prevent fatal hypoglycemia. It is also worth noting that three patients presented with complete refusal of oral feeding secondary to progressive food refusal. Although alternative feeding routes are a necessary resource for some patients with GSD (Rake et al. 2002), tube feeding is known to cause adverse events, including negative impact on the stomatognathic system, and hinder swallowing and feeding behavior (Dunitz-Scheer et al. 2009; Gomes et al. 2015).

The study participants exhibited reduced olfactory and taste perception, and we identified an association between this reduced perception and feeding issues. These findings are consistent with the literature on FDs (Dunitz-Scheer et al. 2009; Edwards et al. 2015; Evans et al. 2017). It is well known that varied sensory experiences in childhood feeding (olfactory, gustatory, and others) play an important role in promoting proper and pleasant eating habits. It is understood that, in GSDs, olfactory and taste perception may be limited by the lack of stimuli caused by the highly restrictive diet, particularly regarding fruits and some vegetables.

We also found a high prevalence of FDs in the sample, which suggests that individuals with GSD have a higher frequency of selective intake and fear of feeding when compared to children without these diseases. Benjasuwantep et al. (2013) reported a 15.4% prevalence of selective intake and 0.25% prevalence of fear of feeding in the general population. Kerzner et al. (2015) and Edwards et al. (2015) note that children with chronic diseases or behavioral issues tend to develop feeding difficulties. In their study of phenylketonuria, an inborn error of metabolism which also requires a restrictive diet for proper management, Evans et al. (2017) showed that neophobia is mainly caused by fear of eating foods that may be forbidden in the patient's diet.

The high frequency of negative eating situations and behaviors identified in this sample corroborates previous studies showing that gastrointestinal abnormalities, orofacial myofunctional disorders, and the use of alternative feeding routes are mechanical and structural aspects that frequently cause feeding difficulty. Family habits and unfavorable and stressful environments have also been described as behavioral factors that predispose to food refusal and selective intake (Dunitz-Scheer et al. 2009; Kerzner et al. 2015; Edwards et al. 2015). Benjasuwantep et al. (2013) reported that children with eating problems tend to eat at the table with their families less often and have prolonged feeding times.

Within this context, we identified that several participants in our sample did not eat meals as a family and found an association between GSD type I and feeding difficulty. These findings may be related to the high overall prevalence of feeding difficulty in the sample, as individuals with feeding problems often do not eat at the family table (Dunitz-Scheer et al. 2009; Benjasuwantep et al. 2013), as well as to the disease itself and its treatment, since patients with hepatic GSD need to eat at prescribed times, which may diverge from family mealtimes (Rake et al. 2002; Weinstein and Wolfsdorf 2002; Flanagan et al. 2015). In the case of GSD type I, dietary control is associated with even greater restrictions and need for even more frequent intake of uncooked cornstarch to maintain normoglycemia and prevent secondary metabolic disorders than in other GSD subtypes (Rake et al. 2002; Flanagan et al. 2015).

In the present sample, the youngest patients and those with feeding difficulties performed worse on the orofacial myofunctional test. This finding is consistent with previous studies describing that structural and mechanical abnormalities, such as OMDs, can cause feeding difficulties (mainly selective intake and food aversion). Refusal of solid or difficult-to-chew foods is usually due to changes in breathing, swallowing, and mastication patterns, as well as aversive behaviors due to gagging, odynophagia, and increased protective oral reflexes (Dunitz-Scheer et al. 2009; Kerzner et al. 2015; Edwards et al. 2015).

We conclude that there is a high prevalence of feeding difficulties and orofacial myofunctional disorders in Brazilian patients with hepatic GSD. Our results suggest that individuals with GSD I subtypes may be at higher risk of feeding disorders and orofacial myofunctional disorders compared to those with other GSD subtypes also requiring strict dietary management. This warrants further evaluation. Likewise, our suspicion of decreased olfactory and taste perception in these patients was confirmed, especially for sourness. Weaknesses of this study include the fact that no validated protocol was used to assess feeding behavior, the small sample size, and the single-center design, which will have influenced dietary treatment practices and the eating habits of patients.

Our results also indicate that individuals with hepatic GSD may be inordinately susceptible to orofacial myofunctional disorders and feeding difficulties, due to factors related to the disease itself, to its treatment, and to eating habits. We suggest that clinicians involved in the management of GSDs need to be alert for selective intake, food refusal, and difficulties in chewing and swallowing in childhood and adulthood, especially in children during the period of food introduction, and should refer patients with these issues to specialist professionals for evaluation and follow-up. Further research on this topic be conducted to confirm whether olfactory and taste perception are reduced in these patients and investigate possible causes for these sensory impairments, as well as to support early identification of eating disorders and feeding difficulties and development of therapeutic interventions to address these issues.

Acknowledgments The authors thank the team of the Medical Genetics Service and the Research and Graduate Program of Hospital de Clínicas de Porto Alegre (HCPA) for the collaboration in this study. We also thank the patients and families of patients with hepatic glycogen storage disease who kindly agreed to participate in this study. CAPES, CNPQ, FAPERGS, and FIPE (HCPA) also supported the work.

Concise One Sentence About Manuscript

Prevalence of feeding difficulties and orofacial myofunctional disorders in patients with hepatic glycogen storage disease.

General Rules

- *Details of the Contributions of Individual Authors*

    Chenia Caldeira Martinez: author took the lead in design project; acquisition, interpretation, and analysis of data; was responsible for the writing of manuscript.

    Tássia Tonon: contributed to the design of study; acquisition, interpretation, and analysis of data; revised the manuscript in order to approve the final version.

    Tatiéle Nalin and Lilia Farret Refosco: both coauthors contributed to the conception and design of study; interpretation and analysis of data; revised critically the article in order to approve the final version of this manuscript.

    Carolina Fischinger Moura de Souza and Ida Vanessa Doederlein Schwartz: both coauthors contributed to the idealization; conception and design of study; interpretation and analysis of data; revised critically the article in order to approve the final version of this manuscript.

- *A Competing Interest Statement*

    Chenia Caldeira Martinez, Tatiéle Nalin, Tássia Tonon, Lilia Farret Refosco, Carolina Fischinger Moura de Souza, and Ida Vanessa Doederlein Schwartz declare that they have no conflict of interest.

- *Details of Funding*

    Project funded by Fundo de Incentivo à Pesquisa e Eventos (FIPE) of Hospital de Clínicas de Porto Alegre.

- *Details of Ethics Approval*

    The study was approved by the Research Ethics Committee of Hospital de Clínicas de Porto Alegre (protocol no. 150072).

- *A Patient Consent Statement*

    According to the project no. 150072 of Ethics Committee of Hospital de Clínicas de Porto Alegre, a written informed consent was obtained from all individuals before participation in the study.

- *Documentation of Approval from the Institutional Committee for Care and Use of Laboratory Animals (or Comparable Committee)*

References

Benjasuwantep B, Chaithirayanon S, Eiamudomkan M (2013) Feeding problems in healthy young children: prevalence, related factors and feeding practices. Pediatr Rep 5(2):38–42

Carruth BR, Ziegler PJ, Gordon A, Barr SI (2004) Prevalence of picky eaters among infants and toddlers and their caregivers' decisions about offering a new food. J Am Diet Assoc 104(1): s57–s64

Chen YT, Kishnani PS (2012) Glycogen Storage Disease and Other Inherited Disorders of Carbohydrate Metabolism. In: Longo DL et al (eds) Harrison's principles of internal medicine, vol II, 18th edn. McGraw-Hill, New York, pp 3198–3203

Chou JY, Matern D, Mansfield BC, Chen YT (2002) Type I glycogen storage diseases: disorders of the glucose-6-phosphatase complex. Curr Mol Med 2(2):121–143

Correia CE et al (2008) Use of modified cornstarch therapy to extend fasting in glycogen storage disease types Ia and Ib. Am J Clin Nutr 88:1272–1276

Dagli A, Sentner CP, Weinstein DA (2016) Glycogen storage disease type III. GeneReview, 2016. https://www.ncbi.nlm.nih.gov/books/NBK26372/. Accessed 16 Jan 2018

De Felício CM, Ferreira CLP (2008) Protocol of orofacial myofunctional evaluation with scores. Int J Pediatr Otorhinolaryngol 7(3):367–375

Derks TG, Smit GP (2015) Dietary management in glycogen storage disease type III: what is the evidence? J Inherit Metab Dis 38 (3):545–550

Dunitz-Scheer M et al (2009) Prevention and treatment of tube dependency in infancy and early childhood. Infant Child Adolesc Nutr 1(2):73–82

Edwards S et al (2015) Interdisciplinary strategies for treating oral aversions in children. JPEN J Parenter Enteral Nutr 39(8):899–909

Evans S, Daly A, Chahal S, Ashmore C, MacDonald J, MacDonald A (2017) The influence of parental food preference and neophobia on children with phenylketonuria (PKU). Mol Genet Metab Rep 14:10–14

Flanagan TB, Sutton JA, Brown LM, Weinstein DA, Merlo LJ (2015) Disordered eating and body esteem among individuals with glycogen storage disease. JIMD Rep 19:23–29

Gomes CA Jr et al (2015) Percutaneous endoscopic gastrostomy versus nasogastric tube feeding for adults with swallowing disturbances. Cochrane Database Syst Rev 5:CD008096

Hummel T, Sekinger B, Wolf SR, Pauli E, Kobal G (1997) 'Sniffin' Sticks': olfactory performance assessed by the combined testing of odor identification, odor discrimination and olfactory threshold. Chem Senses 22(1):39–52

Janecke AR, Mayatepek E, Utermann G (2001) Molecular genetics of type 1 glycogen storage disease. Mol Genet Metab 73(2):117–125

Kerzner B, Milano K, MacLean WC Jr, Berall G, Stuart S, Chatoor I (2015) A practical approach to classifying and managing feeding difficulties. Pediatrics 135(2):344–353

Kishnani PS, Austin SL, Abdenur JE et al (2014) Diagnosis and management of glycogen storage disease type I: a practice guideline of the American College of Medical Genetics and Genomics. Genet Med 16(11):e1–e1

Mascola AJ, Bryson SW, Agras WS (2010) Picky eating during childhood: a longitudinal study to age 11-years. Eat Behav 11(4):253–257

Mueller C et al (2003) Quantitative assessment of gustatory function in a clinical context using impregnated "taste strips". Rhinology 41(1):2–6

Rake JP, Visser G, Labrune P, Leonard JV, Ullrich K, Smit GP (2002) Glycogen storage disease type I: diagnosis, management, clinical course and outcome. Results of the European Study on Glycogen Storage Disease Type I (ESGSD I). Eur J Pediatr 161(l):S20–S34

Santos BL et al (2014) Glycogen storage disease type I: clinical and laboratory profile. J Pediatr 90(6):572–579

Walter J, Labrune P, Laforêt P (2016) The glycogen storage diseases and related disorders. In: Saudubray JM, Baumgartner MR, Walter J (eds) Inborn metabolic diseases: diagnosis and treatment, 6th edn. Springer, Berlin, pp 131–137

Weinstein DA, Wolfsdorf JI (2002) Effect of continuous glucose therapy with uncooked cornstarch on the long-term clinical course of type 1a glycogen storage disease. Eur J Pediatr 161: S35–S39

Wolfsdorf JI, Weinstein DA (2003) Glycogen storage disease. Rev Endocr Metab Disord 4:95–102

Wright CM, Parkinson KN, Shipton D, Drewett RF (2007) How do toddler eating problems relate to their eating behavior, food preferences, and growth? Pediatrics 120(4):e1069–e1075

JIMD Reports
DOI 10.1007/8904_2018_137

RESEARCH REPORT

Auxiliary Partial Orthotopic Liver Transplantation for Monogenic Metabolic Liver Diseases: Single-Centre Experience

Naresh P. Shanmugam · Joseph J. Valamparampil ·
Mettu Srinivas Reddy · Khoula Julenda Al Said ·
Khalid Al-Thihli · Nadia Al-Hashmi ·
Emtithal Al-Jishi · Hasan Mohamed Ali Isa ·
Anil B. Jalan · Mohamed Rela

Received: 08 June 2018 / Revised: 27 July 2018 / Accepted: 20 August 2018 / Published online: 12 October 2018
© Society for the Study of Inborn Errors of Metabolism (SSIEM) 2018

Communicated by: Georg Hoffmann

N. P. Shanmugam · J. J. Valamparampil · M. S. Reddy · M. Rela
Institute of Liver Disease and Transplantation, Gleneagles Global
Health City, Chennai, India
e-mail: drnareshps@gmail.com; josephvalam@yahoo.co.in;
smettu.reddy@gmail.com; mohamed.rela@gmail.com

N. P. Shanmugam · J. J. Valamparampil · M. S. Reddy · M. Rela (✉)
Institute of Liver Disease and Transplantation, Dr. Rela Institute &
Medical Centre, Bharat Institute of Higher Education & Research,
Chennai, India
e-mail: drnareshps@gmail.com; josephvalam@yahoo.co.in;
smettu.reddy@gmail.com; mohamed.rela@gmail.com

K. J. Al Said · N. Al-Hashmi
Royal Hospital, Muscat, Oman
e-mail: drkhoula@gmail.com; nadia.alhashmi@gmail.com

K. Al-Thihli
Genetic and Developmental Medicine Clinic, Sultan Qaboos
University, Muscat, Oman
e-mail: khalid.althihli@gmail.com

E. Al-Jishi
Paediatric and Inborn Error of Metabolism, Salmaniya Medical
Complex, Manama, Bahrain
e-mail: ejishi77@gmail.com

H. M. A. Isa
Salmaniya Medical Complex, Manama, Bahrain
e-mail: halfaraj@hotmail.com

H. M. A. Isa
Arabian Gulf University, Manama, Bahrain
e-mail: halfaraj@hotmail.com

A. B. Jalan
Paediatric and Inborn Error of Metabolism, Navi Mumbai Institute of
Research in Mental and Neurological Handicap, Navi Mumbai, India
e-mail: jalananil12@gmail.com

M. Rela
Institute of Liver Studies, King's College Hospital, London, UK
e-mail: mohamed.rela@gmail.com

Abstract *Purpose*: Auxiliary partial orthotopic liver transplantation (APOLT) in metabolic liver disease (MLD) has the advantage of correcting the metabolic defect, preserving the native liver for gene therapy in the future with the possibility of withdrawal of immunosuppression.

Methods: Retrospective analysis of safety and efficacy of APOLT in correcting the underlying defect and its impact on neurological status of children with MLD.

Results: A total of 13 APOLT procedures were performed for MLD during the study period. The underlying aetiologies being propionic acidemia (PA)-5, citrullinemia type 1 (CIT1)-3 and Crigler-Najjar syndrome type 1 (CN1)-5 cases respectively. Children with PA and CIT1 had a median of 8 and 4 episodes of decompensation per year, respectively, before APOLT and had a mean social developmental quotient (DQ) of 49 ($<$3 standard deviations) as assessed by Vineland Social Maturity Scale prior to liver transplantation. No metabolic decompensation occurred in patients with PA and CIT1 intraoperatively or in the immediate post-transplant period on protein-unrestricted diet. Patients with CN1 were receiving an average 8–15 h of phototherapy per day before APOLT and had normal bilirubin levels without phototherapy on follow-up. We have 100% graft and patient survival at a median follow-up of 32 months. Progressive improvement in neurodevelopment was seen in children within 6 months of therapy with a median social DQ of 90.

Conclusions: APOLT is a safe procedure, which provides good metabolic control and improves the neurodevelopment in children with selected MLD.

Introduction

Auxiliary partial orthotopic liver transplantation (APOLT) is a surgical procedure where a portion of native liver is removed and a partial liver graft is placed in the space created (Reddy et al. 2017; Rela et al. 2016). This is in contrast to standard orthotopic liver transplantation (OLT) where the whole liver is removed and replaced with an allograft. APOLT is an excellent option in selected cases of acute liver failure, where the native liver can regenerate and immunosuppression withdrawn; its utility in metabolic liver disease (MLD) is still being criticized due to complexity of surgical technique and a continued need for immunosuppression (Reddy et al. 2017; Rela et al. 2016). Here, we report our experience with APOLT for selected MLD.

Materials and Methods

Clinical data of children who underwent APOLT for MLD over a period of 9 years (July 2009–May 2018) at Institute of Liver Disease and Transplantation was retrospectively analysed. The criteria for patient selection, operative procedure of APOLT and refinements in operative techniques for APOLT for MLD have been described in detail previously (Reddy et al. 2017; Rela et al. 2013, 2016; Kaibori et al. 1998).

Clinical records of these patients were reviewed to collect the following data: indications for performing APOLT, gender, age at onset, symptoms at presentation, type of feeds, mode of feeding, total number of metabolic decompensations, frequency of hospitalizations, need for invasive ventilation, haemodialysis, pre-transplant neurological status and status of metabolic control prior to transplant. Data was also collected about time from onset of disease to APOLT, ABO-blood-type matching, graft types, graft-to-recipient weight ratio (GRWR), donor demographics, postoperative complications, day of initiation of normal feeds, metabolic decompensations in the post-transplant period, immunosuppressive therapy, incidence of rejection and duration of follow-up.

Primary endpoints were patient survival, graft survival and graft function. Secondary endpoints were the improvement of developmental quotient (DQ), the number of episodes of metabolic decompensation in patients with PA and CIT1 and the need for phototherapy in children with CN1. Developmental status was assessed using developmental screening test (DST) and Vineland Social Maturity Scale (VSMS) prior to and 6 months after APOLT (in PA and CIT1). Disease severity (DS), metabolic status (MS), neurological status (NS) and quality of life were assessed by grading scales used previously to compare children with liver-based metabolic disorder as shown in Table 1 (Morioka et al. 2005a, b).

Table 1 Grading scales to evaluate disease severity, metabolic status and neurological status and classifications of quality of life (used with permission from Morioka et al. 2005a, b)

Severity of the disease (DS):
Grade 4: Many episodes of severe hyperammonemic coma, some with $NH3^a > 300$ µmol/L
Grade 3: One to several episodes of hyperammonemic coma, no more than one with $NH3^a > 300$ µmol/L
Grade 2: One to few episodes of hyperammonemic coma, none with $NH3^a > 300$ µmol/L
Grade 1: Only one episode of hyperammonemic coma, with $NH3^a < 300$ µmol/L
Grade 0: No episodes of hyperammonemic coma, no $NH3^a > 300$ µmol/L

Metabolic status (MS):
Grade 4: No improvement, severe hyperammonemia and need for constant, full doses of medication
Grade 3: Some improvement, moderate hyperammonemia and need for constant medication
Grade 2: Major improvement, moderate hyperammonemia and need for some medication for control
Grade 1: Almost complete correction, occasional hyperammonemia and with or without need for medication
Grade 0: Completer correction, no hyperammonemia and no need for medication

Neurological status (NS):
Grade 5: Persistent coma or vegetative state
Grade 4: Responds to noxious stimuli, but no social interaction, no ambulation and no communication
Grade 3: Limited social interaction, no bipedal ambulation and limited communication through gestures
Grade 2: Definite social interaction and fair ambulation, though possibly limited by spasticity
Grade 1: Good social interaction and full ambulation but perhaps partially impaired gross and fine motor skills and use of language, mildly delayed development and only modest learning deficits
Grade 0: Seems to be normal spectrum for social interaction, motor skills and language development and learning

Quality of life:
Excellent: Receiving one or no immunosuppressive drugs and all the above grading scales corresponding to a score of 0
Good: Receiving two or more immunosuppressive drugs and all the above corresponding to a score of 0
Fair: Regardless of the number of immunosuppressive drugs each patient received, one or more of the above scales corresponding to a scale to 1
Poor: With any episodes of graft dysfunction to necessitate frequent or long hospital stay regardless of their causes and/or one or more of the above scales corresponding to a score of 2 or more

[a] NH3 serum ammonia level, *µmol/L* micromoles/litre

Statistical Methods

Chi-square testing was used to compare categorical variables, while comparisons of continuous variables were performed with the t test and Mann-Whitney U test. SPSS commercial statistics software was used for all statistical analyses (PASW Statistics ver. 18.0; IBM Co., Armonk, NY, USA). The p-values less than 0.05 were considered to be significant. Values were reported as medians and ranges unless stated otherwise.

Results

During the study period, a total of 291 children below 18 years of age underwent liver transplantation (LT), of which 13 APOLT procedures were performed for MLD. The underlying MLD were propionic acidemia (PA) in five, citrullinemia type 1 (CIT1) in three and Crigler-Najjar syndrome type 1 (CN1) in five patients. Details of three patients have been reported previously (Shanmugam et al. 2011; Govil et al. 2015).

Patient Characteristics

Propionic Acidemia ($n = 5$) and Citrullinemia Type 1 ($n = 3$)

These two diseases are grouped together for discussion as both are disorders of amino acid metabolism with elevated ammonia during decompensation and similar medical management during decompensation. The age of presentation ranged from 3 to 6 days after birth, with a median of 3 days. All children with CIT1 and three patients with PA presented with a history of poor feeding, encephalopathy, acidosis and hyperammonemia. Two patients with PA were diagnosed prenatally by genetic assay (patients 2 and 3). Seven patients (58%) had fatal family history due to MLD.

All children with PA and CIT1 were on protein-restricted feeds prior to APOLT. Patients 4 and 8 were on supportive nasogastric feeds. Difficulty in procuring special feeds was a significant concern for Indian patients prior to LT since it had to be imported and was expensive. In the PA subgroup, three were on carglumic acid, two were on sodium benzoate and all received carnitine and biotin, prior to APOLT. All patients with CIT1 were on arginine and sodium benzoate.

Indications for APOLT in PA and CIT1 were frequent metabolic decompensations, poor quality of life, diet restriction and delayed development in all except one. Patient 3 did not have any metabolic decompensation prior to LT and had normal developmental milestones, but parents opted for LT since caring for the child was restricting the quality of life of the parents and siblings.

Patient 1 with PA had dilated left ventricle (LV) with hypokinesia (LV ejection fraction – 45%) and hypertension.

Crigler-Najjar Syndrome Type 1 ($n = 5$)

The median serum bilirubin value prior to transplantation was 393 μmol/L (range 325–496 μmol/L) in spite of 8–15 h of phototherapy daily. Patients 10 and 11 had normal developmental milestones but were taken up for APOLT because it was difficult to restrict children under phototherapy. Patient 9 had normal milestones while on phototherapy but developed bilirubin encephalopathy at the age of 1.5 years during an episode of intercurrent infection. During that episode, he required mechanical ventilation due to refractory seizures, following which he had developmental delay. Patients 12 and 13 had developmental delay with poor social skills.

APOLT Procedure

The age of patients at APOLT ranged from 8 to 264 months, with a median of 32 months. All transplants were performed as left auxiliary liver transplants. Patient 11 with CN1 received a domino auxiliary graft from patient 5 with propionic acidemia (Govil et al. 2015). All patients underwent intraoperative portal flow modulation as previously described (Reddy et al. 2017; Shanmugam et al. 2011; Rela et al. 2015). None of the patients developed portal steal phenomenon in the immediate post-transplant period. The median duration of hospital stay after transplantation was 18 days (range 14–45 days). The pre-/post-APOLT demographics and follow-up data are summarized in Table 2.

Post-transplant Course

The immediate postoperative period was uneventful with no episodes of metabolic or hepatic decompensation in children with PA and CIT1 except for patient 5. All children received total parenteral nutrition for first 3–5 days with 1 g/kg of bodyweight of protein until enteral feeds were started with close monitoring of serum ammonia and amino acid levels. Enteral protein supplements were gradually increased to unrestricted diet over a period of 5 days with monitoring of ammonia. All children were on normal diet/standard formula intake by the 10th postoperative day. Facilitating oral intake was difficult in many children since they were on enteral tube feeds and were not used to the taste and texture of normal diet. Patient 4 was on nasogastric feeds 6 months after APOLT due to feeding difficulties.

The postoperative recovery was uneventful in all patients with CN1. Serum bilirubin levels normalized within 6 days

Table 2 Characteristics of APOLT for metabolic liver disease

Case	Diagnosis	Sex	Metabolic decompensations (per year)	Pre-transplant complications	Age at APOLT (months)	LDLT/DDLT	Type	Graft weight	GRWR	Donor	Follow-up (months)	DQ Pre/post APOLT	Pre-transplant status[a] (DS/MS/NS)	Status at the latest evaluation[a] (DS/MS/NS)	Quality of life at the latest evaluation[a]	Outcome
1	PA	Male	8–10	Mechanical ventilation (twice) Pancytopenia Septicaemia	55	LDLT	LLS	254	1.7	Uncle	50	44/90	4/4/3	0/0/0	Excellent	Alive
2	PA	Male	4–6	Mechanical ventilation (twice) Pancreatitis Septicaemia	21	LDLT	LLS	231	2.1	Father	31	26/65	4/4/2	0/0/0	Excellent	Alive
3	PA	Male	0	Neutropenia	8	LDLT	LLS	191	1.7	Uncle	34	100/100	0/0/0	0/0/0	Excellent	Alive
4	PA	Female	4–5	Developmental delay	33	LDLT	LLS	355	3.9	Mother	19	56/94	4/4/3	0/0/1	Fair	Alive
5	PA	Male	3–4	Developmental delay Seizures Pancytopenia	38	LDLT	LLS (graft reduction)	231	2.3	Mother	36	38/86	4/4/4	0/0/0	Excellent	Alive
6	CIT1	Male	3	Developmental delay Seizures	23	DDLT	LLS	245	2.9	Cadaveric	40	22/68	4/4/3	0/0/1	Fair	Alive
7	CIT1	Female	1	Nil	39	LDLT	LLS	320	3.7	Mother	20	95/105	0/0/1	0/0/0	Excellent	Alive
8	CIT1	Male	2–3	Developmental delay	32	DDLT	LLS	233	2.6	Cadaveric	19	54/90	4/4/3	0/0/0	Excellent	Alive
9	CN1	Male	NA	Developmental delay Extrapyramidal syndrome	22	LDLT	LLS (graft reduction)	233	2.6	Mother	13	85/100	NA/NA/4	NA/NA/1	Fair	Alive
10	CN1	Female	NA	Nil	26	LDLT	LLS	248	2.4	Mother	21	Not available	NA/NA/0	NA/NA/0	Excellent	Alive
11	CN1	Male	NA	Nil	49	LDLT	Left lobe	233	2.3	Domino auxiliary from patient 5	36	100/100	NA/NA/0	NA/NA/0	Excellent	Alive
12	CN1	Female	NA	Cerebellar involvement Speech delay	264	DDLT	LLS	385	2.6	Cadaveric	99	100/100	NA/NA/1	NA/NA/1	Fair	Alive
13	CN1	Male	NA	Speech delay, hyperactivity	96	LDLT	LLS	247	0.47	Mother	5	Not available	NA/NA/0	NA/NA/0	Excellent	Alive

PA propionic acidemia, *CIT1* citrullinemia type I, *CN1* Crigler-Najjar syndrome type 1, *NA* not applicable, *APOLT* auxiliary partial orthotopic liver transplantation, *LDLT* living donor liver transplantation, *DDLT* deceased donor liver transplantation, *LLS* left lateral segment, *GRWR* graft-to-recipient weight ratio (%), *DQ* developmental quotient, *DS* disease severity, *MS* metabolic status, *NS* neurological status

[a] Assessed by grading scales or classified into subgroups as shown in Table 1 (used with permission from reference) Morioka et al. 2005a, b

after APOLT (range 3–7 days), and none of the children required phototherapy after surgery.

Immunosuppression Post-APOLT

All patients were on standard immunosuppression with tacrolimus and steroids as per our unit protocol. Trough tacrolimus levels were maintained between 10 and 12 nanogram/millilitre (ng/mL) in first 3 months, 8–10 ng/mL for next 6 months and 5–7 ng/mL later on. Steroids were started at 2 mg/kg and then tapered to 1 mg/day (same dose for all patients) over the next 3 weeks. Children were monitored for rejection based on aminotransferase level elevation. Any elevated levels were evaluated with tacrolimus level, Doppler ultrasound to evaluate preferential graft portal perfusion and biopsy of the native and graft liver. Rejection confirmed by biopsy was treated with intravenous methyl prednisolone for 3–5 days followed by oral taper to 1 mg/day.

Post-transplant Complications

Four children had six episodes of histologically proven steroid-responsive acute cellular rejection. The first episode of rejection occurred after a median of 35 days (range 22–70 days). Patient 5 had two more episodes of steroid-responsive rejection 114 days and 180 days after APOLT. None of the rejection episodes were associated with metabolic decompensation.

One child with PA (patient 5) was diagnosed with hepatic artery thrombosis on the 6th postoperative day. He underwent immediate surgical revascularization and made a complete recovery. Over a follow-up period of 30 months, his graft function remains good.

Patient 3 with PA had an episode of high ammonia without encephalopathy during an episode of intercurrent illness 9 months after APOLT. A segmental portal vein embolization of the native liver was performed to cause segmental atrophy of the native liver and facilitate compensatory hypertrophy of the graft. This rapidly corrected the metabolic abnormality, and the child has remained asymptomatic without further episodes of decompensations with good graft function over 29 months of follow-up.

Patient 8 with CIT1 developed gastrointestinal post-transplant lymphoproliferative disorder 6 months after APOLT. He was managed with immunosuppression withdrawal and rituximab. There were no episodes of rejection or metabolic decompensation during the time period. He recovered well, immunosuppression was reintroduced 6 months later and he is presently on regular follow-up with good graft function and disease in remission.

Follow-Up

We have 100% graft and patient survival at a mean follow-up of 32 months (range 5–99 months). All children with PA and CIT1 had metabolic cure of hyperammonemia and are on unrestricted diets. Carnitine supplementation was stopped in patient 1 resulting in low serum-free carnitine and elevated acyl carnitine levels and so was restarted. All other children with PA were continued on carnitine and biotin supplementation. Cardiomyopathy and hypertension in patient 1 did not progress after liver transplantation, and the patient has remained stable on follow-up of 50 months. He continues to take digoxin for cardiac problem and lisinopril for hypertension.

All three children with CIT1 had serum citrulline levels of more than 2,000 μmol/L before transplant that has reduced to 300–800 μmol/L after transplant on a median follow-up of 20 months. CIT1 patients continued to receive arginine supplementation. CN1 patients have normal bilirubin values without phototherapy.

Development and Quality of Life

Patients with PA and CIT1 had a mean social developmental quotient (DQ) of 49 (<3 standard deviation) as assessed by VSMS prior to APOLT. Progressive improvement in developmental scores was seen in children within 6 months of therapy with a median social DQ of 90. Disease severity, metabolic status, neurological status and quality of life prior to APOLT and at the last follow-up are shown in Table 2.

Discussion

Metabolic liver diseases are a group of liver-based monogenic inherited disorders that cause disruption in normal metabolic pathways due to the absence of specific protein, which could be an enzyme or a receptor (Fagiuoli et al. 2013; Sokal 2006). MLD could be grossly divided into cirrhotic and non-cirrhotic (Fagiuoli et al. 2013; Sokal 2006). Non-cirrhotic could be further divided into those with primary defective hepatic enzyme expression, such as CN1, or defective hepatic and extrahepatic expression such as PA and CIT1 (Fagiuoli et al. 2013).

APOLT is primarily indicated in non-cirrhotic MLD where the gene defect leads to a deficiency or lack of a specific enzyme or protein such as CN1, urea cycle defects, etc. (Reddy et al. 2017). APOLT should not be offered in cirrhotic metabolic disorders as there is a potential risk of development of malignancy in the remnant native liver (Reddy et al. 2017). This procedure is also not recommended for MLD such as primary hyperoxaluria and primary hypercholesterolemia where an excess of toxic substrates such as oxalate crystals and cholesterol, respectively, are produced (Reddy et al. 2017; Trotter and Milliner 2014). The retained native liver in primary hyperoxaluria will continue to produce oxalate crystals, which will continue to damage the kidneys, while continued production of cholesterol in primary hypercholesterolemia would result in progressive atherosclerosis (Reddy et al. 2017; Trotter and Milliner 2014).

APOLT in the setting of LT for MLD has several distinct advantages. Most MLD need only small amount of enzyme activity to be completely symptom-free. This could range from 20% for PA to just around 5% for CN1 (Fagiuoli et al. 2013). Replacing an entire, otherwise normal liver in these children is unnecessary. A small graft is usually sufficient for these patients; hence, a split left lateral segment may be sufficient even for an adult, while a smaller graft can improve donor safety in the setting of LDLT. Since there is no need for a total hepatectomy during APOLT, the stress of the anhepatic phase and the risk of intraoperative metabolic crises are sharply reduced. APOLT also decreases the cardiac stress associated with LT (Blankensteijn et al. 1990). In MLD with defective hepatic and extrahepatic expression, whether OLT or APOLT, there is only partial correction of the defect, and in theory, these children could have metabolic crisis during an intercurrent illness (Baba et al. 2016).

Domino liver transplantation involves the use of a genetically defective liver as a graft for a second recipient and can be used in the setting of MLD when the extrahepatic organs of the recipient are able to compensate for the deficient gene in the allograft liver (example: maple syrup urine disease). We have expanded this concept further and used liver graft from a child with PA in a child with CN1 (Govil et al. 2015). Patient can survive with two hemilivers, each with a different metabolic defect without clinical or biochemical manifestation, because each genetically defective hemiliver cancels the metabolic defect of the other (Govil et al. 2015).

Domino liver transplantation between MLD patients requires a basic understanding of the disease pathology and the complications. For example, it is not feasible for primary hyperoxaluria liver to be used as domino graft because the allograft will continue to produce oxalate which will damage the recipient's kidneys and could lead to renal failure (Popescu and Dima 2012). The other important considerations include the informed consent of both the domino recipient and the donor, compatible blood groups and size-matched liver grafts.

Living donor liver transplantation with heterozygous donors has been documented to be safe and effective in CN1, CIT1 and PA (Morioka et al. 2005a, b). The effectiveness of genetic evaluation in MLD other than ornithine transcarbamylase deficiency is uncertain (Morioka et al. 2005a, b). In a large series of LT for MLD, neither mortality nor morbidity related to the heterozygous state was observed for the recipient or the donor (Morioka et al. 2005a, b). No differences were noted between the cadaveric and related grafts in our study. Based on the analysis of data from a large group of urea cycle disorder patients who underwent LDLT, it has been postulated that neurological impairment is more likely to remain in deceased donor LT than in those who underwent LDLT, but the difference was not of statistical significance (Morioka et al. 2005a, b).

None of the children with PA and CIT1 in our series had intraoperative or perioperative decompensation necessitating the need for dialysis (Baba et al. 2016). The highest recorded ammonia and lactate were 76 μmol/L and 2.2 mmol/L, respectively, during intraoperative period. APOLT provides intraoperative and perioperative stability as there is no anhepatic phase during surgery, potentially eliminating the risk of metabolic crisis during the time period in these disorders (Fagiuoli et al. 2013). Carnitine supplementation in PA and arginine in CIT1 is indicated even after transplantation, the reason being allograft donor liver is the only source of missing enzyme, while the metabolic defect continues to persist in the rest of the body.

In CN1, high unconjugated bilirubin fraction can cross the blood-brain barrier and damage the brain, resulting in neurological sequelae. CN1 requires intense phototherapy for 12–16 h a day to keep unconjugated bilirubin under danger levels. As these children get older, the efficiency of phototherapy declines due to increase in thickness of the skin and increased mobility. Restriction under constant phototherapy affects the quality of life and interferes with the attainment of normal developmental milestones.

Allograft dysfunction due to any cause such as rejection, surgical complications, etc. after OLT could present with metabolic crises and liver failure which could be life-threatening and difficult to manage. On the contrary, graft problems in APOLT manifest as a metabolic crisis which can be medically managed as the native liver would support the liver function.

Technical complications including portal steal with early graft dysfunction and long-term graft atrophy have been a major problem with this operation previously (Kasahara et al. 2005). LFT or even disease-specific markers may not be sufficient to diagnose graft atrophy at an early stage (Reddy et al. 2017). We perform 6 monthly Doppler ultrasound to confirm preferential graft portal perfusion in all patients on follow-up. Volumetric computed tomography (CT) to quantify the graft and native liver volume was done 6 monthly in the first year of follow-up and then as per clinical indication. Recurrence of original symptoms in patient 3 was evaluated with Doppler ultrasound, volumetric CT, graft and native liver biopsy.

With technical refinements and careful intraoperative portal flow modulation, this is uncommon as evidenced in our present series (Reddy et al. 2017; Rela et al. 2015, 2016). Sze et al. also reported outcome of APOLT in 11 children with metabolic disease, with no significant difference in patient or graft survival when compared with standard OLT at 1-, 5- and 7-year follow-up (Sze et al. 2009).

Finally, APOLT preserves a part of the patient's native liver for future gene therapy. While this goal may take decades to achieve, it is important to note that most patients undergoing LT for MLD now are small children and will still benefit immensely as young adults from an immunosuppression-free life when gene therapy becomes available.

APOLT is a safe procedure in selective cases of MLD providing adequate metabolic control with improvement in developmental and neurological state. Apart from the added benefit of preserved native liver, it provides greater intra-operative and postoperative stability due to the absence of anhepatic phase during LT. This study shows that APOLT provides adequate metabolic control in selected MLD.

Synopsis

Auxiliary partial orthotopic liver transplantation provides good metabolic control and improves the neurodevelopment in children with selected metabolic liver diseases while retaining a part of the native liver for future gene therapy.

Compliance with Ethics Guidelines

Conflict of Interest

Naresh P. Shanmugam, Joseph J. Valamparampil, Khoula Julenda Al Said, Khalid Al-Thihli, Nadia Al-Hashmi, Emtithal Al-Jishi, Hasan Mohamed Ali Isa, Anil B. Jalan and Mohammed Rela declare that they have no conflict of interest.

Informed Consent

All procedures followed were in accordance with the ethical standards of the responsible committee on human experimentation (institutional and national) and with the Helsinki Declaration of 1975, as revised in 2000 (5). Informed consent was obtained from all patients for being included in the study.

This article does not contain any studies with animal subjects performed by the any of the authors.

Contributions of Individual Authors

Naresh P. Shanmugam and Joseph J. Valamparampil – collection of clinical information, literature review and manuscript writing. Khoula Julenda Al Said, Khalid Al-Thihli, Nadia Al-Hashmi, Emtithal Al-Jishi, Hasan Mohamed Ali Isa and Anil B. Jalan – literature review and review of manuscript. Prof. Mohammed Rela oversaw all aspects of the manuscript preparation and edited the manuscript. Prof. Mohamed Rela will be the guarantor for the article.

References

Baba C, Kasahara M, Kogure Y, Kasuya S, Ito S, Tamura T (2016) Perioperative management of living-donor liver transplantation for methylmalonic acidemia. Paediatr Anaesth 26:694–702

Blankensteijn JD, Groenland TH, Baumgartner D, Vos LP, Kerkhofs LG, Terpstra OT (1990) Intraoperative hemodynamics in liver transplantation comparing orthotopic with heterotopic transplantation in the pig. Transplantation 49:665–668

Fagiuoli S, Daina E, D'Antiga L, Colledan M, Remuzzi G (2013) Monogenic diseases that can be cured by liver transplantation. J Hepatol 59:595–612

Govil S, Shanmugam NP, Reddy MS, Narasimhan G, Rela M (2015) A metabolic chimera: two defective genotypes make a normal phenotype. Liver Transpl 21:1453–1454

Kaibori M, Egawa H, Inomata Y et al (1998) Selective portal blood flow diversion in auxiliary partial orthotopic liver transplantation to induce regeneration of the graft. Transplantation 66:935–937

Kasahara M, Takada Y, Egawa H, Fujimoto Y, Ogura Y, Ogawa K (2005) Auxiliary partial orthotopic living donor liver transplantation: Kyoto University experience. Am J Transplant 5:558–565

Morioka D, Kasahara M, Takada Y et al (2005a) Current role of liver transplantation for the treatment of urea cycle disorders: a review of the worldwide English literature and 13 cases at Kyoto University. Liver Transpl 11:1332–1342

Morioka D, Kasahara M, Takada Y et al (2005b) Living donor liver transplantation for pediatric patients with inheritable metabolic disorders. Am J Transplant 5:2754–2763

Popescu I, Dima SO (2012) Domino liver transplantation: how far can we push the paradigm? Liver Transpl 18:22–28

Reddy MS, Rajalingam R, Rela M (2017) Revisiting APOLT for metabolic liver disease: a new look at an old idea. Transplantation 101:260–266

Rela M, Bharathan A, Rajalingam R, Narasimhan G, Reddy MS (2013) Technique of hepatic arterial anastomosis in living donor pediatric auxiliary partial orthotopic liver transplantation. Liver Transpl 19:1046–1048

Rela M, Bharathan A, Palaniappan K, Cherian PT, Reddy MS (2015) Portal flow modulation in auxiliary partial orthotopic liver transplantation. Pediatr Transplant 19:255–260

Rela M, Kaliamoorthy I, Reddy MS (2016) Current status of auxiliary partial orthotopic liver transplantation for acute liver failure. Liver Transpl 22:1265–1274

Shanmugam NP, Perumalla R, Gopinath R, Olithselvan A, Varghese J, Kapoor D (2011) Auxiliary liver transplantation: a form of gene therapy in selective metabolic disorders. J Clin Exp Hepatol 1:118–120

Sokal EM (2006) Liver transplantation for inborn errors of liver metabolism. J Inherit Metab Dis 29:426–430

Sze YK, Dhawan A, Taylor RM, Bansal S, Mieli-Vergani G, Rela M, Heaton N (2009) Paediatric liver transplantation for metabolic liver disease: experience at King's College Hospital. Transplantation 87:87–93

Trotter JF, Milliner D (2014) Auxiliary liver transplant is an ineffective treatment of primary hyperoxaluria. Am J Transplant 14:241

JIMD Reports
DOI 10.1007/8904_2018_139

RESEARCH REPORT

A Novel Truncating *FLAD1* Variant, Causing Multiple Acyl-CoA Dehydrogenase Deficiency (MADD) in an 8-Year-Old Boy

B. Ryder · M. Tolomeo · Z. Nochi · M. Colella ·
M. Barile · R. K. Olsen · M. Inbar-Feigenberg

Received: 14 April 2018 / Revised: 15 August 2018 / Accepted: 20 August 2018 / Published online: 12 October 2018
© Society for the Study of Inborn Errors of Metabolism (SSIEM) 2018

Abstract Multiple acyl-CoA dehydrogenase deficiency (MADD) or glutaric aciduria type II (GAII) is a clinically heterogeneous disorder affecting fatty acid and amino acid metabolism. Presentations range from a severe neonatal form with hypoglycemia, metabolic acidosis, and hepatomegaly with or without congenital anomalies to later-onset lipid storage myopathy. Genetic testing for MADD traditionally comprises analysis of *ETFA*, *ETFB*, and *ETFDH*. Patients may respond to pharmacological doses of riboflavin, particularly those with late-onset MADD due to variants in *ETFDH*. Increasingly other genes involved in riboflavin transport and flavoprotein biosynthesis are recognized as causing a MADD phenotype. Flavin adenine dinucleotide synthase (FADS) deficiency caused by biallelic variants in *FLAD1* has been identified in nine previous cases of MADD. *FLAD1* missense mutations have been associated with a riboflavin-responsive phenotype; however the effect of riboflavin with biallelic loss of function *FLAD1* mutations required further investigation. Herein we describe a novel, truncating variant in *FLAD1* causing MADD in an 8-year-old boy. Fibroblast studies showed a dramatic reduction in FADS protein with corresponding reduction in the FAD synthesis rate and FAD cellular content, beyond that previously documented in *FLAD1*-related MADD. There was apparent biochemical and clinical response to riboflavin treatment, beyond that previously reported in cases of biallelic loss of function variants in *FLAD1*. Early riboflavin treatment may have attenuated an otherwise severe phenotype.

M. Barile and R. K. Olsen contributed equally to this work.

Communicated by: Piero Rinaldo, MD, PhD

Electronic supplementary material: The online version of this chapter (https://doi.org/10.1007/8904_2018_139) contains supplementary material, which is available to authorized users.

B. Ryder · M. Inbar-Feigenberg
Division of Clinical and Metabolic Genetics, The Hospital for Sick Children, University of Toronto, Toronto, ON, Canada

B. Ryder (✉)
National Metabolic Service, Starship Children's Hospital, Auckland, New Zealand
e-mail: bryonykryder@gmail.com

M. Tolomeo · M. Colella · M. Barile
Department of Bioscience, Biotechnology and Biopharmaceutics, University of Bari, Bari, Italy

Z. Nochi · R. K. Olsen
Research Unit for Molecular Medicine, Department for Clinical Medicine, Aarhus University and Aarhus University Hospital, Aarhus, Denmark

Introduction

Multiple acyl-CoA dehydrogenase deficiency (MADD, MIM #231680) or glutaric aciduria type II is an autosomal recessive disorder causing defective electron transport from flavin adenine dinucleotide (FAD)-containing dehydrogenases to coenzyme Q10 in the mitochondrial electron transport chain. The condition is clinically heterogeneous ranging from a severe, neonatal form, presenting with hypoketotic hypoglycemia, metabolic acidosis, cardiomyopathy, and hepatomegaly to a later-onset form characterized by proximal myopathy. The neonatal form is further subdivided based on the presence of congenital anomalies including dysplastic kidneys, cerebral malformations, pulmonary hypoplasia, facial dysmorphism, and abnormal genitalia (Grünert 2014). Episodic vomiting, encephalopathy, liver and renal impairment, rhabdomyolysis, and sudden death may occur at times of catabolic stress (Horvath 2012).

Plasma acylcarnitine profile findings of elevated short-, medium- and long-chain acylcarnitines (C4–C16) may be diagnostic or absent if carnitine depleted (Wen et al. 2015). Urine organic acid analysis may show increased ethylmalonic acid, 2-hydroxyglutarate, glutaric acid, lactate, dicarboxylic acids, and glycine conjugates. Creatine phosphokinase (CPK) and lactate levels are typically raised during metabolic decompensation. Biochemical findings may normalize during periods of stability. Muscle biopsy reveals lipid accumulation in skeletal muscle and reduced activity of mitochondrial respiratory chain complexes I + III and II + III and coenzyme Q10 (Vergani et al. 1999; Olsen et al. 2007; Horvath 2012).

Genetic changes in *ETFA* (15q23-q25) and *ETFB* (19q13.3-q13.4) encoding the alpha and beta subunits of electron transport flavoprotein (ETF) and *ETFDH* (4q32-q35) encoding ETF-ubiquinone oxidoreductase (ETFQO), respectively, were first identified as causing MADD. *ETFDH* variants are the most common cause of late-onset disease (Grünert 2014). Both ETF and ETFOQ contain FAD prosthetic groups (Henriques et al. 2010). Deficiencies in FAD therefore inhibit activity of ETF and ETFOQ as well as other FAD-dependent enzymes, causing MADD.

Riboflavin (vitamin B2), the precursor for flavin mononucleotide (FMN) and FAD, cannot be synthesized in humans. It is consumed in dietary sources such as meat and dairy, absorbed in the intestine, transported into the blood stream, and taken up by one of three tissue-specific riboflavin transporters thus far identified (RFVT 1, 2, 3), encoded by *SLC52A1*, *SLC52A2*, and *SLC52A3* (Barile et al. 2016). Inside the cell, riboflavin kinase converts riboflavin into FMN, which is adenylated to FAD, by FAD synthase (FADS), encoded by *FLAD1* (Brizio et al. 2006). Activated FADS may chaperone the folding of apoproteins into stable flavoproteins (Giancaspero et al. 2015).

Biochemical features of MADD have been noted in newborns of mothers with riboflavin deficiency and heterozygous mutations in *SLC52A1* (Chiong et al. 2007; Ho et al. 2011) and in patients with Brown–Vialetto–Van Laere (BVVL) syndrome, caused by mutations in *SLC52A2* or *SLC52A3* (Haack et al. 2012). More recently, mutations in the mitochondrial FAD transporter gene (*SLC25A32*, MIM 610815) (Schiff et al. 2016) and FAD synthase gene (*FLAD1*, MIM 610595) (Olsen et al. 2016) have been shown to cause MADD. While *FLAD1* missense mutations were associated with a riboflavin-responsive phenotype, the effect of riboflavin with biallelic loss of function *FLAD1* mutations was less clearly defined. Herein we describe a novel, truncating variant in *FLAD1* causing riboflavin-responsive MADD myopathy in an 8-year-old boy.

Case Report

The patient was referred to the metabolic service with a positive newborn screen for medium-chain acyl-CoA dehydrogenase (MCAD) deficiency, due to an elevated C8-acylcarnitine of 0.58 µM (<0.4). He was the first child to consanguineous, first cousins of Palestinian descent. The antenatal history was unremarkable, and he was born by normal vaginal delivery at 40-week gestation, with a birth weight of 3.268 kg. No resuscitation was required, and he fed well 3 h, on a combination of breast milk and formula. Family history was noncontributory and examination normal. The diagnosis of MADD was made when a confirmatory plasma acylcarnitine profile detected elevations in C6–C10 acylcarnitines and urine organic acid analysis detected ethylmalonic acid, 2-hydroxyglutaric acid, glutaric acid, and dicarboxylic aciduria (for biochemical results, see Supplementary Material). Other blood work was normal, including liver enzymes and CPK. Riboflavin (10 mg/kg/day) was initiated at 16 days of age. No pathogenic variants were identified in *ETFA*, *ETFB*, or *ETFDH* (Emory Genetics). An elevated CPK (457) was noted at 3 months of age during his first hospital admission and recurred with subsequent recurrent respiratory infections. Riboflavin was increased to 50 mg/kg/day and carnitine added (100 mg/kg/day). Dietary fat was restricted from 48% of calories from fat at baseline to 32%; however a fat- and protein-restricted diet has never been closely adhered to. Riboflavin was stopped at 29 months of age due to low palatability, while carnitine was continued. A myopathic open mouth appearance was first noted at aged 3 years with nasal speech and open mouth breathing not improved following tonsillectomy and adenoidectomy. On otorhinolaryngology review, aged 6 years, he had hypernasality, weak facial muscles, and a wet cough. The palate did not elevate on phonation, and he displayed significant oral incoordination. Laryngoscopy identified severe velopharyngeal insufficiency, and a wide surgical velopharyngeal flap was recommended.

By 8 years of age, he had an evolving myopathy with fatigue on chewing and worsening exercise intolerance. He was achieving normally in mainstream schooling. Hearing tests performed in the community were normal. He had not attended for ophthalmology review. Annual cardiac evaluation including echocardiogram and electrocardiogram (ECG) were normal. Height was on the 25th centile (122.3 cm) and weight on the 10th (20.5 kg). He had myopathic facies with a tented downturned mouth held in an open position. Dental caries affected the upper dentition, and he had a high-arched palate with no visible cleft. There was no facial asymmetry, and he was able to protrude his tongue in the midline but was unable to raise his eyebrows. Speech was almost unintelligible due to velopharyngeal insufficiency. He had minimal muscle bulk, and tone was generally reduced. Power appeared normal in all four limbs, but reflexes were not obtainable despite reinforcement. Plantars were down-going bilaterally, and there was no clonus. Cardiac, respiratory, and abdominal examinations were all normal.

A microarray identified significant loss of heterozygosity (LOH), consistent with parental consanguinity. The gene for FAD synthase, *FLAD1*, was noted to be within one such region, and targeted sequencing of *FLAD1* identified homozygosity for c.745C > T (p. Arg249*). This nonsense variant results in a premature STOP codon in exon 2 of the molybdopterin-binding (MPTb) domain and is predicted pathogenic (Giancaspero et al. 2015). The variant is seen six times in a heterozygous state but has not previously been reported in the homozygous state (http://gnomad.broadinstitute.org/gene/ENSG00000160688). Functional analyses were performed to better characterize the novel variant. Riboflavin was restarted at 150 mg/day.

Methods

Cell Culturing

Dermal fibroblast cultures from the patient (P) and three healthy, age- and gender-matched controls (C1, C2, C3) (Cambrex #CC-2509, ATCC #CRL-2450, and private donation from Dr. L. Vergani, University of Padua) were incubated at 37°C and humidified atmosphere of 5% (v/v) CO_2 in EMEM (Eagle's minimum essential medium) (Lonza, Basel, Switzerland) supplemented with 2 mmol/L of L-glutamine (Sigma Aldrich, St. Louis, Missouri, USA), 10% fetal calf serum (Sigma Aldrich, St. Louis, Missouri, USA), and 1% penicillin/streptomycin (Sigma Aldrich, St. Louis, Missouri, USA). Following pre-culturing, the cell cultures were transferred to 1×75 cm^2 culture flask and harvested at sub-confluence by detaching in trypsin-EDTA solution, PBS (pH 7.4), centrifuged for 3 min at $405 \times g$, and washed twice in PBS. Fibroblast pellets were stored at $-80°C$ after removal of PBS.

Quantification of Cellular Flavin Content and Measurement of FAD Synthesis Rate

Cell pellets were resuspended in 100 μL lysis buffer (50 mmol/L Tris–HCl [pH 7.5], 1% Triton X-100, 5 mmol/L ß-mercaptoethanol [2-ME], 1 mmol/L NaF, 0.1 mmol/L PMSF, and 1 x protease inhibitor cocktail) and passed through a 26G needle. After incubation for 30 min on ice, the cell suspension was centrifuged at $13,000 \times g$ for 10 min at 4°C, and the supernatant was recovered as cell lysate. Protein content was determined by the Bradford protein assay (Bio-Rad, Hercules, California,

USA). Riboflavin, FMN, and FAD were measured in neutralized perchloric acid extracts of cell lysates (0.2 mg) by HPLC as previously described (Liuzzi et al. 2012).

The rate of FAD synthesis was measured at 37°C in 600 μL of 50 mM Tris–HCl (pH 7.5) in the presence of 0.2 mg cell lysate, 1 μmol/L FMN, 5 mmol/L ATP, and 5 mmol/L $MgCl_2$. At the appropriate time, 100 μL aliquots were taken, extracted with perchloric acid, and neutralized. Quantitative determination of riboflavin, FMN, and FAD was carried out with a calibration curve made in each experiment with standard solutions diluted in the extraction solution.

Western Blotting

Frozen cell pellets were dissolved in lysis buffer on ice (50 mM Tris–HCl pH 7.8, 5 mM EDTA, 1 mM DTT, 1% Triton X-100, and one protease inhibitor cocktail tablet (cOmplete Mini, Roche, Mannheim, Germany) in 10 mL), followed by 30 s of sonication in ultrasonic bath (Bandelin SONOREX™ SUPER with built-in heating ultrasonic baths) (Sigma Aldrich, St. Louis, Missouri, USA). The lysate was separated into Triton X-100 soluble and insoluble fractions by 15 min of centrifugation at $14,800 \times g$, 4°C.

20 and 40 μg of the total cell protein extract [determined by the Bradford protein assay (Bio-Rad, Hercules, California, USA)] were analyzed by SDS-PAGE on Criterion™ TGX Stain-free™ Precast Gels (any kD) (Bio-Rad, Hercules, California, USA) in Tris-glycine 0.1% SDS buffer. All Blue Standards (Bio-Rad, Hercules, California, USA) was used as molecular weight (MW) marker. Proteins were blotted onto PVDF membranes [midi format, 0.2 μm (Bio-Rad, Hercules, California, USA)] by semidry electro-blotting [Trans-Blot® Turbo™ Transfer System (Bio-Rad, Hercules, California, USA)] for 30 min. The PVDF membranes were incubated 1 h in 5% nonfat skim milk (VWR, Radnor, Pennsylvania, USA). Transferred proteins were incubated overnight with primary polyclonal rabbit antibodies: (1) anti-VLCAD (very long-chain Acyl-CoA dehydrogenase) antibody (kindly provided by Dr. Arnie Strauss), diluted 1:10,000 (detected at MW 68 kDa); (2) anti-SCAD (short-chain acyl-CoA dehydrogenase) antibody (kindly provided by Dr. Kay Tanaka), diluted 1:15,000 (detected at MW 40 kDa); (3) anti-ETF A and B (electron transfer flavoprotein α and β) antibody (kindly provided by Dr. Kay Tanaka) diluted 1:20,000 (detected at MW 32 and 27 kDa); and (4) anti-FLAD1 antibody (HPA028563) (Sigma Aldrich, St. Louis, Missouri, USA), diluted 1:250 (detected at MW 54 kDa). Polyclonal goat anti-rabbit-HRP antibody (DAKO, Copenhagen, Denmark) at dilution 1:20,000 was used as secondary antibody. ECL plus Western blotting detection system (Amersham Biosciences,

Little Chalfont, UK) was used for protein detection, according to manufacturer's recommendations. Detection was done using the ImageQuant LAS 4000 (GE Healthcare, Little Chalfont, UK). The intensities of bands were quantified using ImageQuant TL (GE Healthcare, Little Chalfont, UK) and normalized to total protein content.

Results

Flavin Content and FAD Synthesis Rate in Fibroblasts

The rate of FAD synthesis in cultured fibroblast from the affected individual was drastically reduced with respect to the control range (0.35 pmol/min mg *versus* 3.50–4.37 pmol/min mg, student's t-test $p < 0.001$) (Fig. 1). FAD synthesis impairment resulted in a significant reduction in FAD content (Table 1) measured in cultured fibroblasts from the affected individual (60.5 pmol/mg, student's t-test $p < 0.05$) with respect to that found from controls (ranging from 111.7 to 171.2 pmol/mg). Quite surprisingly, there was also a significant reduction in the cellular content of FMN (5.8 pmol/mg, student's t-test $p < 0.001$) and riboflavin (1.0 pmol/mg, student's t-test $p < 0.01$) to 44 and to 33%, respectively, that of control

values, suggesting a regulatory metabolic response to FADS impairment.

FADS and Flavoenzyme Protein Levels in Fibroblasts

FADS and flavoenzyme protein levels in patient and control fibroblasts were determined by Western blot analysis. As expected from the *FLAD1* genotype, the MADD patient fibroblasts displayed significantly decreased full-length 50 kDa FADS protein levels compared to control fibroblasts (student's t-test $p < 0.001$). However, the 26 kDa FADS band, which was suggested to contain an intact and functional FADS domain (Olsen et al. 2016), seems equally expressed in both patient and control fibroblasts (Fig. 2a, b). Mitochondrial flavoproteins comprising very long-chain acyl-CoA dehydrogenase (VLCAD), short-chain acyl-CoA dehydrogenase (SCAD), and the two ETF subunit proteins showed a tendency to be decreased in the patient as compared to control, although neither of the results was statistically significant (Fig. 3a, b).

Discussion

This is the tenth published case of MADD due to biallelic pathogenic variants in *FLAD1*. The age of onset in the nine

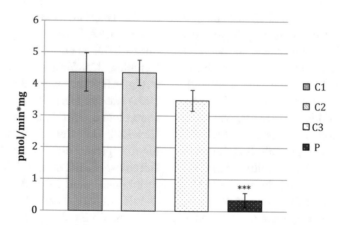

Fig. 1 The rate of FAD synthesis was measured in fibroblasts from the patient (P) and from three control individuals (C1, C2, and C3), as described in Sect. 3. Data represent the mean ± SD of two independent cell lysates; student's t-test: ***$p < 0.001$

Table 1 Cellular FAD, FMN, and riboflavin quantification in fibroblast samples

Cellular flavin content (pmol/mg)

	FAD	FMN	Rf
C1	111.7 ± 2.8	13.3 ± 1.4	2.6 ± 0.5
C2	171.2 ± 18.8	12.4 ± 0.3	3.1 ± 0.1
C3	123.3 ± 15.1	14.3 ± 1.3	3.5 ± 0.6
P	60.5 ± 2.6*	5.8 ± 1.1***	1.0 ± 0.4**

For cellular flavin content, data represent the mean ± SD of two independent cell lysates; student's t-test: *$p<0.05$, **$p<0.01$, and ***$p<0.001$

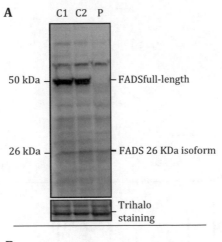

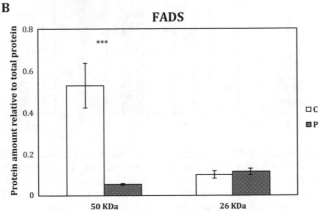

Fig. 2 (**a**) Representative immunoblot analysis of FADS protein. Protein extracts from cultured human dermal fibroblasts were separated by SDS-PAGE and immunoblotted with a polyclonal antibody, raised against the C-terminal part of human FAD synthase protein (FADS). The patient cells were cultured in two separate cultures together with two healthy control individuals (C1 and C2); protein was extracted and 40 μg loaded on Criterion™ TGX Stain-free™ Precast Gels (any kD) (Bio-Rad). The molecular weight of protein bands identified as FADS by mass spectrometry analysis (Olsen et al. 2016) is indicated. (**b**) FADS protein intensities were quantified relative to total protein content (Trihalo staining). Quantification of patient FADS relative to combined two control individuals as shown. The error bars represent standard error of mean (SEM) of two independent experiments, student's *t*-test: ***$p < 0.001$

previously reported cases of *FLAD1*-related MADD ranges from birth to 44 years, however most presented in infancy, with five out of nine dying in the first year of life (Taylor et al. 2014; Olsen et al. 2016). A lipid storage myopathy with respiratory chain deficiency predominates, similar to *ETFDH*-related riboflavin-responsive forms of MADD. Cardiomyopathy has been reported once, and two patients required pacemaker insertion for tachyarrhythmia/cardiac arrest (Olsen et al. 2016). Neuropathies, hearing or visual impairment as seen in BVVL (Bosch 2011), have not yet been described with *FLAD1* variants. Hypotonia, swallowing, and speech difficulties as seen in this case are typical (Olsen et al. 2016).

Two major human *FLAD1* transcript products, FADS1 (mitochondrial) and FADS2 (cytosolic), have been characterized in detail (Brizio et al. 2006; Barile et al. 2016); however, only the cytosolic isoform was identified in human fibroblasts (Olsen et al. 2016). FADS contains an N-terminal molybdopterin-binding (MPTb) domain with FAD hydrolase activity and a C-terminal domain, which catalyzes FAD synthesis (FADS domain) (Giancaspero et al. 2015). Patients with biallelic frameshift variants in exon 2, i.e., in the MPTb domain, as found in our case, have had early-onset, severe disease (Olsen et al. 2016).

Consistently, fibroblast studies in our patient revealed a dramatic reduction in FADS protein level with corresponding reduction in both FAD synthesis rate and FAD cellular content. Previous studies measuring residual FADS activity in individuals with *FLAD1* variants revealed only a partial defect in FAD synthesis ability of affected fibroblasts, with corresponding cellular FAD, FMN, and riboflavin content within the control range. A low mitochondrial FAD content was observed in one patient (Olsen et al. 2016). While the previously observed residual FAD synthesis activity could be explained by missense mutations in some cases, even previous cases of biallelic frameshift

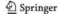

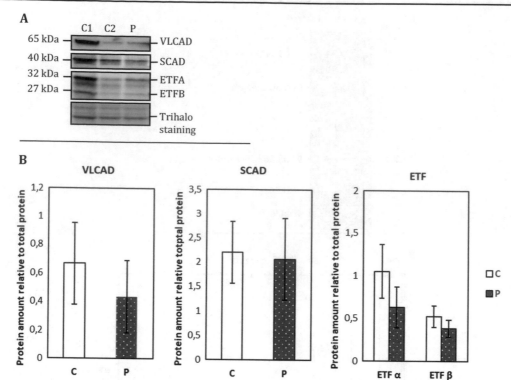

Fig. 3 (a) Representative immunoblot analysis of ACAD proteins. Protein extracts from cultured human dermal fibroblasts were loaded in 20 μg. Samples were separated by SDS-PAGE and immunoblotted with polyclonal antibodies raised against each of the four mitochondrial flavoproteins VLCAD, SCAD, or the two ETF subunit proteins. The patient cells were cultured in two separate cultures together with two healthy control individuals (C1 and C2); protein was extracted and loaded on Criterion™ TGX Stain-free™ Precast Gels (any kD) (Bio-Rad). (b) Protein intensities were quantified relative to total protein content (Trihalo staining). Quantification of patient FADS relative to combined two control individuals as shown. The error bars represent standard error of mean (SEM) of two independent experiments. There was no significant difference in the mitochondrial flavoprotein content between patient and control fibroblasts

variants in exon 2 in the MPTb domain, predicted to result in complete loss of function, had some expression of FADS. Since the FADS domain can function independently from the MPTb domain to catalyze FAD synthesis (Miccolis et al. 2012), the authors hypothesized that the residual FADS activity could result from the expression of novel *FLAD1* isoforms coding for the FADS domain alone (Olsen et al. 2016). It was recently confirmed that one of these truncated isoforms, isoform 6, could produce FAD (Leone et al. 2018). While immunoblotting showed almost no detectable full-length FADS in our case, a 26 kDa protein band, corresponding to a truncated FADS protein, is expressed (Fig. 2). The rate of FAD synthesis in our patient's fibroblasts, however, was lower than that measured before, only 9% of controls (Fig. 1) as compared to 25% of controls in a previous case with biallelic frameshift *FLAD1* variants (Olsen et al. 2016). However, cellular content of FAD was only reduced to 54% that of controls (Table 1). There was a minor, but not significant, decrease in mitochondrial flavoproteins VLCAD, ETF-alpha, and ETF-beta (Fig. 3). It is difficult to relate the

significant reduction in FAD synthesis to the milder clinical outcome. FADS activity of 9% that of controls seems to allow cellular FAD supply comparable to heterozygous levels. It is likely that FADS is not the rate-limiting step in this process and that residual synthetic activity, possibly complemented by the 26 kDa truncated FADS protein, is sufficiently active to synthesize half of normal total FAD content. The 26 kDa isoform does not contain a mitochondrial leader peptide; therefore mitochondrial FAD supply in patients with biallelic exon 2 loss of function mutations depends on import by the mitochondrial FAD transporter. This may become limiting during periods of catabolic stress, when the expression of mitochondrial flavoproteins is increased. The clinical course may have been modified by treatment with riboflavin from the neonatal period until 2.5 years of age, and he may have maintained adequate general health and caloric intake, such as to avoid significant catabolic stress.

It should be noted that in our patient's fibroblasts, there was also an unexpected reduction in the cellular content of FMN and riboflavin rather than the expected increase in substrate levels before the enzymatic block at FADS. A reduction of FAD associated with a reduction of FMN and riboflavin has been also found in the model organism *C. elegans* with silenced FAD synthase gene (Liuzzi et al. 2012). Feedback control on either riboflavin kinase or SLC52A2/RFVT2 was proposed but has not yet been documented. It is possible that either the riboflavin kinase or the riboflavin transporter step is the rate-limiting step in FAD synthesis overall process, and a secondary deficiency may result from disturbed flavin homeostasis, causing reduced FMN synthesis or riboflavin transport. No reported cases of riboflavin kinase deficiency in humans have yet been described.

Flavoproteins, such as mitochondrial acyl-CoA dehydrogenases, appear to undergo rapid degradation in a state of riboflavin deficiency (Henriques et al. 2010). A trial of high-dose riboflavin supplementation (100–400 mg/day) is recommended in all MADD cases. Riboflavin has low toxicity even at high doses as riboflavin exceeding renal reabsorption is eliminated in the urine (Barile et al. 2016). Side effects are largely limited to non-specific gastrointestinal disturbance. Riboflavin responsiveness has been reported in *FLAD1* variants, more often in milder variants affecting a single amino acid in the FADS domain (Auranen et al. 2017). Four out of five patients treated showed a response, including improved cardiac and skeletal muscle function, normalization of urinary organic acids, and reductions in acylcarnitine species (Olsen et al. 2016). Patients with biallelic frameshift variants in exon 2 were more severely affected and less responsive to riboflavin therapy. Based on plasma acylcarnitine profiles and urine organic acid excretion, our patient did appear to partially respond to riboflavin. Off riboflavin his acylcarnitine profile showed more widespread and higher elevations in acylcarnitine species, and urine organic acids showed excretion of ethylmalonic acid (EMA), 2-hydroxyglutaric, glutaric, adipic, and suberic acids. On riboflavin, only urine EMA was detected. Urine EMA on riboflavin was 30% that of urine EMA excretion off riboflavin (see Supplementary Material). Once treatment with 150 mg/day of riboflavin was restarted, his parents reported better muscle endurance and ability to chew food although this has not been quantified objectively.

In summary, this report describes the clinical, biochemical, and molecular findings of an 8-year-old boy with *FLAD1*-related MADD. Newborn screening was positive for MCAD deficiency, although the pattern was atypical and diagnostic evaluation identified MADD. Disorders of riboflavin metabolism must be considered in the differential diagnosis for MADD to ensure prompt treatment. Although commenced in the neonatal period, riboflavin treatment was not adhered to, and myopathic symptoms became evident by 4 years of age. Recent discovery of homozygous frameshift variants in *FLAD1* has been clinically significant as it has provided the necessary motivation for compliance with riboflavin therapy. Fibroblast studies have shown a dramatic reduction in FADS protein with corresponding reduction in FAD synthesis rate and FAD cellular content, beyond that previously documented in *FLAD1*-related MADD. The presence of biallelic truncating mutations with a significant reduction in cellular flavin content predicts a severe, potentially lethal phenotype. This may have been prevented by early treatment with riboflavin, myopathy developing when riboflavin was ceased, or by relative avoidance of catabolic stress. The residual synthetic activity, possibly complemented by the 26 kDa truncated FADS protein, seems to be sufficient to allow for mitochondrial flavoprotein biogenesis, except at times of catabolic stress. Further studies are planned to clarify the feedback mechanism controlling cellular flavin content.

Key Message

Analysis of *FLAD1* is recommended in cases of MADD, if no pathological variants are identified in *ETFA*, *ETFB*, or *ETFDH*, and a trial of riboflavin is recommended in all patients with *FLAD1* variants.

Author Contributions

Ryder B: primary drafting of the manuscript and clinical care of patient.

Tolomeo M: scientist performing quantification of cellular flavin content and measurement of FAD synthesis rate.

Nochi Z: scientist performing Western blot analysis of FADS and flavoenzymes.

Colella M: senior scientist supervising cell culturing and management.

Barile M: senior scientist supervising quantification of cellular flavin content and measurement of FAD synthesis rate.

Olsen R: senior scientist supervising Western blot analysis of FADS and flavoenzymes.

Inbar-Feigenberg M: primary metabolic physician directing patient care, senior clinician supervising drafting of manuscript.

Corresponding Author

Dr. Bryony Ryder

Conflict of Interest

No conflicts of interest reported.

Acknowledgments and Funding

The study was supported by the Danish Council of Independent Medical Research grant (4004-00548) to Olsen RK.

M. Tolomeo was supported by a postgraduate research fellowship financed by "Fondazione Cassa di Risparmio di Puglia," Bari, Italy.

The technical assistance in HPLC measurements of Dr. M.L. Defrancesco (University of Bari) and in immunoblotting to Margrethe Kjeldsen is gratefully acknowledged.

Thanks to Stacy Hewson and Michelle Mecija for their clinical care.

Compliance with Ethical Standards

Ethics approval was not required for this paper.

Parental consent was obtained for the publication of the article.

This article does not contain any studies with human or animal subjects performed by the any of the authors.

References

Auranen M et al (2017) Patient with multiple acyl-CoA dehydrogenation deficiency disease and *FLAD1* mutations benefits from riboflavin therapy. Neuromuscul Disord 27:581–584

Barile M et al (2016) Riboflavin transport and metabolism in humans. J Inherit Metab Dis 39(4):545–557

Bosch AM (2011) Brown-Vialetto-Van Laere and Fazio Londe syndrome is associated with a riboflavin transporter defect mimicking mild MADD: a new inborn error of metabolism with potential treatment. J Inherit Metab Dis 34(1):159–164

Brizio C et al (2006) Over-expression in Escherichia coli and characterization of two recombinant isoforms of human FAD synthetase. Biochem Biophys Res Commun 344(3):1008–1016

Chiong MA et al (2007) Transient multiple acyl-CoA dehydrogenation deficiency in a newborn female caused by maternal riboflavin deficiency. Mol Genet Metab 92:109–114

Fu HX et al (2016) Significant clinical heterogeneity with similar ETFDH genotype in three Chinese patients with late-onset multiple acyl-CoA dehydrogenase deficiency. Neurol Sci 37 (7):1099–1105

Giancaspero TA et al (2015) Human FAD synthase is a bi-functional enzyme with a FAD hydrolase activity in the molybdopterin binding domain. Biochem Biophys Res Commun 465 (3):443–449

Grünert S (2014) Clinical and genetical heterogeneity of late-onset multiple coenzyme A dehydrogenase deficiency. Orphanet J Rare Dis 9:117

Haack TB et al (2012) Impaired riboflavin transport due to missense mutations in SLC52A2 causes Brown-Vialetto-Van Laere syndrome. J Inherit Metab Dis 35(6):943–948

Henriques BJ, Olsen RK, Bross P, Gomes CM (2010) Emerging roles for riboflavin in functional rescue of mitochondrial β-oxidation flavoenzymes. Curr Med Chem 17(32):3842–3854

Ho G et al (2011) Maternal riboflavin deficiency, resulting in transient neonatal-onset glutaric aciduria Type 2, is caused by a microdeletion in the riboflavin transporter gene GPR172B. Hum Mutat 32(1):E1976–E1984

Horvath R (2012) Update on clinical aspects and treatment of selected vitamin responsive disorders II (riboflavin and CoQ10). J Inherit Metab Dis 35(4):679–687

Leone P et al (2018) Bacterial production, characterization and protein modeling of a novel monofunctional isoform of FAD synthase in humans: an emergency protein? Molecules 23(116)

Liuzzi V et al (2012) Silencing of FAD synthase gene in Caenorhabditis elegans upsets protein homeostasis and impacts on complex behavioural patterns. Biochim Biophys Acta 1820:521–531

Miccolis A et al (2012) Bacterial over-expression and purification of the 3′phosphoadenosine 5′phosphosulfate (PAPS) reductase domain of human FAD synthase: functional characterization and homology modelling. Int J Mol Sci 13(12):16880–16898

Olsen R et al (2007) *ETFDH* mutations as a major cause of riboflavin responsive multiple acyl-CoA dehydrogenation deficiency. Brain 130(8):2045–2054

Olsen R et al (2016) Riboflavin-responsive and -non-responsive mutations in FAD synthase cause multiple Acyl-CoA dehydrogenase and combined respiratory chain deficiency. Am J Hum Genet 98:1130–1145

Schiff M et al (2016) SLC25A32 mutations and riboflavin-responsive exercise intolerance. N Engl J Med 374(8):795–797

Taylor R, Pyle A, Griffin H (2014) Use of whole-exome sequencing to determine the genetic basis of multiple mitochondrial respiratory chain complex deficiencies. JAMA 312(1):68–77

Vergani L et al (1999) Riboflavin therapy. Biochemical heterogeneity in two adult lipid storage myopathies. Brain 122(Pt 12):2401–2411

Wen B et al (2015) Multiple acyl-CoA dehydrogenation deficiency as decreased acylcarnitine profile in serum. Neurol Sci 36 (6):853–859. www.omim.org/entry/231680? search=231680&highlight=231680

JIMD Reports
DOI 10.1007/8904_2018_140

RESEARCH REPORT

The Effect of Continuous Intravenous Glucagon on Glucose Requirements in Infants with Congenital Hyperinsulinism

Colin P. Hawkes · Juan J. Lado · Stephanie Givler ·
Diva D. De Leon

Received: 19 June 2018 / Revised: 17 August 2018 / Accepted: 28 August 2018 / Published online: 12 October 2018
© Society for the Study of Inborn Errors of Metabolism (SSIEM) 2018

Abstract *Background/Aims*: Continuous intravenous glucagon is frequently used in the management of severe congenital hyperinsulinism (HI), but its efficacy in these patients has not been systematically evaluated. The aim of this study was to describe the use of continuous intravenous glucagon and to evaluate its effect on the glucose infusion rate (GIR) requirement in infants with HI.

Methods: Retrospective chart review of children with HI who received continuous intravenous glucagon for prevention of hypoglycemia at the Children's Hospital of Philadelphia between 2003 and 2013.

Results: Forty (22 male) infants were included, and median (IQR) age at glucagon treatment was 29 (23, 54) days. Median glucagon dose was 205 (178, 235) mcg/kg/day and duration of treatment was 5 (3, 9) days. GIR reduced from 18.5 (12.9, 22.8) to 11 (6.6, 17.5) mg/kg/min 24 h after starting glucagon ($p < 0.001$), and hypoglycemia frequency reduced from 1.9 (1.3, 2.9) to 0.7 (0.3, 1.2) episodes per day. Vomiting ($n = 11$, 13%), rash ($n = 2$, 2%), and respiratory distress ($n = 15$, 19%) were seen during glucagon treatment.

Colin P. Hawkes and Juan J. Lado contributed equally to this work.

Communicated by: Gerard T. Berry, M.D.

C. P. Hawkes · S. Givler · D. D. De Leon (✉)
Division of Endocrinology and Diabetes, The Children's Hospital of Philadelphia, Philadelphia, PA, USA
e-mail: deleon@email.chop.edu

C. P. Hawkes · D. D. De Leon
Department of Pediatrics, Perelman School of Medicine, University of Pennsylvania, Philadelphia, PA, USA

J. J. Lado
Division of Pediatric Endocrinology, Ann & Robert H Lurie Children's Hospital of Chicago, Chicago, IL, USA

Conclusion: An intravenous glucagon infusion reduces the required GIR to maintain euglycemia, decreasing the risks associated with the administration of high fluid volume or fluids with high-glucose concentrations.

Abbreviations

GIR   Glucose infusion rate
HI   Hyperinsulinism
K_{ATP} ATP-sensitive potassium channel

Introduction

Congenital hyperinsulinism (HI) is a common cause of persistent hypoglycemia in infants and children. This condition is characterized by dysregulated insulin secretion, and delayed treatment is associated with severe hypoglycemia with increased risk of seizures, developmental delay, and permanent brain injury (Palladino and Stanley 2011; Meissner et al. 2003; Steinkrauss et al. 2005; Lord et al. 2015). Causal mutations in eleven genes have been described in congenital HI, with the most severe forms of disease seen in individuals with inactivating mutations affecting the ATP-sensitive potassium channel (K_{ATP}) (Vajravelu and De Leon 2018). However, approximately 50% of infants with congenital HI do not have an identified genetic cause of disease (Lord et al. 2013; Lord and De Leon 2013).

Available medical treatments for the management of infants with HI are limited. Currently, two medications are routinely used to suppress insulin secretion and ameliorate hypoglycemia in these infants: diazoxide, a K_{ATP} channel activator that maintains the channel in the open state, and octreotide, a somatostatin analog (Lord and De Leon 2013). For children with severe HI, medical management can be ineffective in preventing hypoglycemia and pancreatectomy may be required (Lord et al. 2013). Prior to pancreatectomy, these children require a continuous glucose infusion at high concentrations and often at high fluid volumes. Central venous access may be required to deliver high concentrations of intravenous dextrose, which may be associated with increased risk of infection and intestinal ischemia (Hawkes et al. 2016; Barrington 2000). Increased intravenous fluid volumes in neonates can result in fluid overload and cardiac failure, which can also be exacerbated by diazoxide administration (Lord and De Leon 2013). Glucagon is often used to reduce glucose demands and consequently can reduce these risks in infants with congenital HI (Palladino and Stanley 2011; Lord et al. 2013).

Glucagon opposes insulin action (Quesada et al. 2008) and prevents hypoglycemia by stimulating hepatic gluconeogenesis and glycogenolysis, as well as inhibiting glycogen synthesis and hepatic glucose uptake. Glucagon can also stimulate the uptake of amino acids in the liver as well as increase the release of glycerol from adipocytes, both of which can be used for gluconeogenesis [reviewed in (Unger and Cherrington 2012)]. Despite widespread use of intravenous glucagon in congenital HI, the only published reports describing its use have been in neonates with unspecified hypoglycemia (Charsha et al. 2003; Miralles et al. 2002; Carter et al. 1988). There have been concerns raised regarding a possible association between glucagon treatment and thrombocytopenia or hyponatremia (Belik et al. 2001), but thrombocytopenia was not seen in these retrospective studies including 108 infants, and hyponatremia was considered to be related to excess fluid administration (Charsha et al. 2003; Miralles et al. 2002; Carter et al. 1988).

The aim of this study was to determine the effect of intravenous glucagon on the required glucose infusion rate (GIR) in infants with severe HI awaiting surgical management of their disease. As a secondary outcome, we sought to describe the rates of adverse events seen in infants during glucagon infusion.

Methods

A retrospective chart review of infants with HI who were treated with a continuous intravenous glucagon infusion prior to partial or subtotal pancreatectomy between January 2003 and December 2013 at the Children's Hospital of Philadelphia was conducted. The Institutional Review Board at The Children's Hospital of Philadelphia approved this study.

All infants with a diagnosis of focal or diffuse HI who subsequently underwent pancreatic surgery were eligible for inclusion in this study if they were under 6 months of age at the time of glucagon treatment, they received glucagon for greater than 24 h, and glucose measurements in the 24 h prior to glucagon treatment were available. All children treated with glucagon, regardless of age and availability of glucose measurements, were included in the analysis of adverse events during glucagon treatment.

The diagnosis of HI was based on biochemical evidence of insulin excess at the time of plasma glucose <50 mg/dL, as previously described (Ferrara et al. 2016). The time of glucagon initiation was extracted from the electronic health record. Capillary glucose concentrations were monitored during glucagon treatment at least every 3 h, using a point-of-care glucose meter [Lifescan Sure-Step Pro (Johnson & Johnson, PA, USA) prior to 2012 and Nova StatStrip (Novo Nordisk, Bagsvaerd, Denmark) after 2012].

Glucagon Administration

Glucagon was administered intravenously, either through a peripheral or a central intravenous line. For administration, glucagon was diluted in 5% dextrose to a concentration of 42 mcg/mL. The initial dose for all patients was 1 mg in 24 h, independent of body weight. To prevent precipitation, bags of diluted glucagon and infusion tubing were replaced with freshly prepared glucagon every 24 h.

Statistical Analysis

In analyzing the efficacy of glucagon infusion, the primary outcome was the GIR at 24 h before and after starting glucagon infusion. Secondary outcomes were the frequency of hypoglycemia (plasma glucose <70 mg/dL) and hyperglycemia (plasma glucose >140 mg/dL) in the days prior to and during glucagon treatment. The number of hypo- and hyperglycemia events was averaged for up to 4 days before and during glucagon treatment. Non-normally distributed continuous variables including GIR, hypoglycemia frequency, and hyperglycemia frequency before and during treatment were described using medians and interquartile ranges (IQR) and compared using Wilcoxon signed-rank test. Statistical analyses were performed using SPSS 22.0 (IBM, N.Y., USA). Figures were generated using Prism 5.0 (GraphPad Software Inc., California, USA) and Adobe Illustrator 16.0 (Adobe Systems Inc., California, USA).

Results

Eighty-seven children diagnosed with congenital HI were treated with continuous intravenous glucagon infusion prior to pancreatectomy at the Children's Hospital of Philadelphia between January 2003 and December 2013. Of these, 40 were eligible for inclusion in the analysis of glucagon efficacy (7 were over 6 months of age, 31 commenced treatment with glucagon prior to transfer to our center, and 9 were treated with glucagon immediately on admission and did not have 24 h of glucose measurements available prior to treatment with glucagon). All 87 infants were included in the analysis of adverse events during glucagon treatment.

Efficacy of Glucagon Infusion in Children with Congenital HI

Of the 87 infants treated with intravenous glucagon, 40 had data available of glycemic control before and after glucagon treatment. The median (IQR) age at the time of starting glucagon treatment was 29 (23, 56) days of age, and duration of glucagon treatment was 5 (3, 9) days. Demographic and clinical data for these infants are shown in Table 1.

Of the 40 eligible children, 34 had a decreased glucose infusion rate (GIR) 24 h after starting glucagon treatment. Four children had an increased GIR, and two had no change. Intravenous glucose was completely stopped in two infants after starting glucagon. Overall, there was a statistically significant reduction in the median (IQR) GIR during the 24 h following initiation of continuous glucagon infusion compared to 24 h before initiation (18.5 (12.9, 22.8) to 11 (6.6, 17.5) mg/kg/min, $p < 0.001$) (Fig. 1). Starting glucagon was also associated with a reduction in the median (IQR) frequency of hypoglycemia (1.9 (1.3, 2.9) to 0.7 (0.3, 1.2) episodes per day, $p < 0.001$) (Fig. 2a) without a change in the frequency of hyperglycemia (0.8 (0.3, 1.9) to 1 (0.5, 1.7) episodes per day, $p = 0.3$) (Fig. 2b).

Adverse Events

Thirty-five of the 87 children (41%) treated with continuous glucagon infusion experienced adverse events during treatment. Multiple adverse events were reported during treatment. Vomiting ($n = 11$, 13%), rash ($n = 2$, 2%), and respiratory distress ($n = 15$, 19%) are reported side effects of glucagon treatment and were seen in these patients. One patient had thrombocytopenia prior to starting glucagon treatment, but no patient developed thrombocytopenia during glucagon treatment.

Discussion

Continuous intravenous glucagon is effective in the acute management of infants with congenital HI. We have shown

Table 1 Demographics and clinical characteristics

Characteristic	$n = 40$
Male	22 (55%)
Gestational age, weeks	38 (36, 39)
Age at starting glucagon, days	29 (23, 54)
Duration of glucagon treatment, days	5 (3, 9)
Glucagon dose, mcg/kg/day	205 (178, 235)
Concomitant medications	
Diazoxide[a]	0 (0%)
Octreotide	2 (5%)
Genetic mutations	
ABCC8	
Monoallelic	18 (45%)
Biallelic	15 (37.5%)
KCNJ11	
Monoallelic	3 (7.5%)
Biallelic	2 (5%)
None identified	2 (5%)
Pancreatic histology	
Diffuse	24 (60%)
Focal	14 (35%)
Other	2 (5%)

[a] All infants had failed a trial of diazoxide treatment prior to starting glucagon treatment

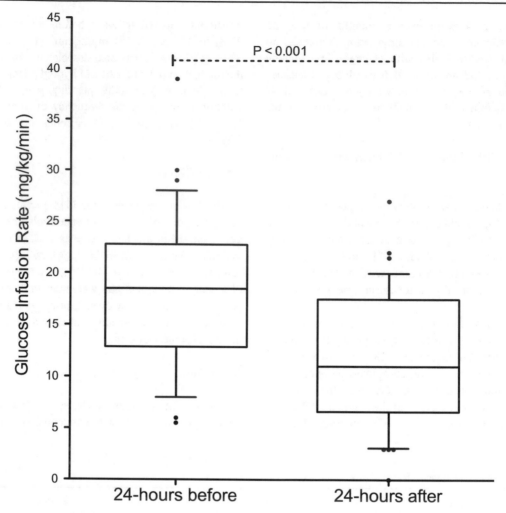

Fig. 1 Glucose infusion rate (GIR, in mg/kg/min) in children with congenital hyperinsulinism 24 h prior to and 24 h after starting continuous glucagon infusion. Box represents 25th and 75th percentiles, and whiskers represent 10th and 90th percentiles

that this treatment is associated with a median reduction in GIR of 7.5 mg/kg/min within 24 h of starting treatment and a significant reduction in the frequency of hypoglycemia without an increase in hyperglycemia. This reduction in GIR can reduce the need for hyperosmolar concentrated glucose or high-volume intravenous infusions. Although numerous adverse events were seen during glucagon treatment, it is not possible to determine if these are related to glucagon infusion, and we generally believe that this is a safe treatment in this population.

When compared with previous studies of glucagon infusion in infants with hypoglycemia, we have observed similar reductions in GIR and hypoglycemia during treatment. However, our study is the first to describe this only in infants with severe HI requiring surgical management. These infants are at particularly high risk of unfavorable developmental outcomes due to the severe and persistent hypoglycemia and often require extremely high concentrations of infused glucose to maintain eugly-

cemia. In infants with congenital HI, endogenous glucagon secretion is blunted during hypoglycemia (Hussain et al. 2005), making exogenous replacement a physiologically appropriate treatment.

There have been concerns regarding the association between treatment of neonates with intravenous glucagon and the development of complications including hyponatremia and thrombocytopenia (Charsha et al. 2003; Miralles et al. 2002; Belik et al. 2001). In this study, we have evaluated the safety of glucagon infusion in the largest reported cohort of treated infants with HI. Only one child in this study had thrombocytopenia, but this was present prior to the initiation of glucagon infusion. Hyponatremia was not seen in any infant included in this study. Vomiting, rash, and respiratory distress are reported adverse effects that may be associated with glucagon administration (Food and Drug Administration n.d.) and, while these were seen in some of the patients included in this study, it is difficult to ascertain that this was associated with glucagon treatment.

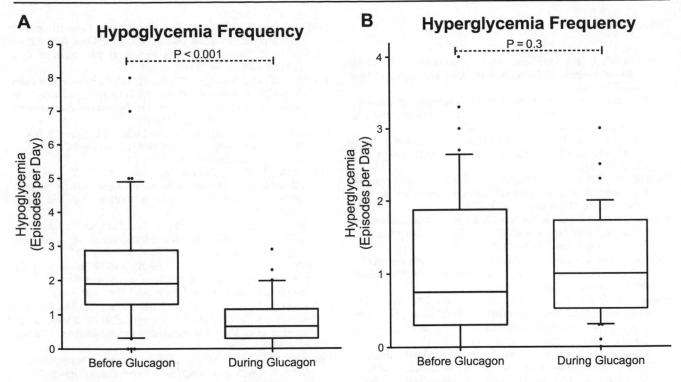

Fig. 2 Frequency of (**a**) hypoglycemia episodes (plasma glucose <70 mg/dL) and (**b**) hyperglycemia episodes (plasma glucose >140 mg/dL) per day in children with congenital hyperinsulinism up to 4 days prior to and 4 days after starting continuous glucagon infusion. Data presented as median (range)

The large number of infants included in this study provides an opportunity to describe the effect of glucagon administration in this patient population and to observe the safety of this treatment. This study is limited by its retrospective design and absence of a control group for comparison. However, by describing only infants who were scheduled for surgical management of their HI, only infants with severe disease and high risk of hypoglycemia were included. Although it is conceivable that GIR prior to starting glucagon may have been unnecessarily high due to insufficient weaning of intravenous glucose, this is unlikely. The frequency of episodes of hypoglycemic was higher prior to starting glucagon, suggesting that it was not possible to wean the GIR further prior to glucagon treatment.

In conclusion, this study demonstrates that continuous glucagon infusion is an effective treatment in severe congenital HI. Starting a glucagon infusion allows for a reduction in GIR in most infants, which will facilitate a reduction in intravenous volume and/or glucose concentration administered. Furthermore, we have not demonstrated significant safety concerns in using glucagon but recommend close observation as these infants are at risk of complications due to their underlying disease, high fluid requirements, and coexisting medications.

Funding Sources

This study was supported by training grant T32DK063688-13S to J.J.L. and grant 5R01DK098517 to D.D.D.L.

Compliance with Ethics Guidelines

All procedures followed were in accordance with the ethical standards of the responsible committee on human experimentation (institutional and national) and with the Helsinki Declaration of 1975, as revised in 2000 (5).

Conflict of Interest

Colin Hawkes, Juan Lado, Stephanie Givler, and Diva D. De Leon declare that they have no conflict of interest.

Author Contributions

Colin Hawkes analyzed data and wrote the manuscript, Juan Lado collected and analyzed data and wrote the manuscript, Stephanie Givler collected data, and Diva D. De Leon designed study and edited the manuscript.

References

Barrington KJ (2000) Umbilical artery catheters in the newborn: effects of position of the catheter tip. Cochrane Database Syst Rev. CD000505

Belik J, Musey J, Trussell RA (2001) Continuous infusion of glucagon induces severe hyponatremia and thrombocytopenia in a premature neonate. Pediatrics 107:595–597

Carter PE, Lloyd DJ, Duffty P (1988) Glucagon for hypoglycaemia in infants small for gestational age. Arch Dis Child 63:1264–1266

Charsha DS, McKinley PS, Whitfield JM (2003) Glucagon infusion for treatment of hypoglycemia: efficacy and safety in sick, preterm infants. Pediatrics 111:220–221

Ferrara C, Patel P, Becker S, Stanley CA, Kelly A (2016) Biomarkers of insulin for the diagnosis of hyperinsulinemic hypoglycemia in infants and children. J Pediatr 168:212–219

Food and Drug Administration (n.d.) Glucagon for injection (rDNA origin). https://www.accessdata.fda.gov/drugsatfda_docs/label/2015/201849s002lbl.pdf

Hawkes CP, Adzick NS, Palladino AA, De Leon DD (2016) Late presentation of fulminant necrotizing enterocolitis in a child with hyperinsulinism on octreotide therapy. Horm Res Paediatr 86 (2):131–136

Hussain K, Bryan J, Christesen HT, Brusgaard K, Aguilar-Bryan L (2005) Serum glucagon counterregulatory hormonal response to hypoglycemia is blunted in congenital hyperinsulinism. Diabetes 54:2946–2951

Lord K, De Leon DD (2013) Monogenic hyperinsulinemic hypoglycemia: current insights into the pathogenesis and management. Int J Pediatr Endocrinol 2013:3

Lord K, Dzata E, Snider KE, Gallagher PR, De Leon DD (2013) Clinical presentation and management of children with diffuse and focal hyperinsulinism: a review of 223 cases. J Clin Endocrinol Metab 98:E1786–E1789

Lord K, Radcliffe J, Gallagher PR, Adzick NS, Stanley CA, De Leon DD (2015) High risk of diabetes and neurobehavioral deficits in individuals with surgically treated hyperinsulinism. J Clin Endocrinol Metab 100(11):4133–4139

Meissner T, Wendel U, Burgard P, Schaetzle S, Mayatepek E (2003) Long-term follow-up of 114 patients with congenital hyperinsulinism. Eur J Endocrinol 149:43–51

Miralles RE, Lodha A, Perlman M, Moore AM (2002) Experience with intravenous glucagon infusions as a treatment for resistant neonatal hypoglycemia. Arch Pediatr Adolesc Med 156:999–1004

Palladino AA, Stanley CA (2011) A specialized team approach to diagnosis and medical versus surgical treatment of infants with congenital hyperinsulinism. Semin Pediatr Surg 20:32–37

Quesada I, Tuduri E, Ripoll C, Nadal A (2008) Physiology of the pancreatic alpha-cell and glucagon secretion: role in glucose homeostasis and diabetes. J Endocrinol 199:5–19

Steinkrauss L, Lipman TH, Hendell CD, Gerdes M, Thornton PS, Stanley CA (2005) Effects of hypoglycemia on developmental outcome in children with congenital hyperinsulinism. J Pediatr Nurs 20:109–118

Unger RH, Cherrington AD (2012) Glucagonocentric restructuring of diabetes: a pathophysiologic and therapeutic makeover. J Clin Invest 122:4–12

Vajravelu ME, De Leon DD (2018) Genetic characteristics of patients with congenital hyperinsulinism. Curr Opin Pediatr 30 (4):568–575

JIMD Reports
DOI 10.1007/8904_2018_142

RESEARCH REPORT

Case of Neonatal Fatality from Neuromuscular Variant of Glycogen Storage Disease Type IV

Tavleen Sandhu · Michelle Polan · Zhongxin Yu · Rufei Lu · Abhishek Makkar

Received: 15 June 2018 / Revised: 06 August 2018 / Accepted: 10 September 2018 / Published online: 12 October 2018
© Society for the Study of Inborn Errors of Metabolism (SSIEM) 2018

Abstract Glycogen storage disease type IV (GSD-IV), or Andersen disease, is a rare autosomal recessive disorder that results from the deficiency of glycogen branching enzyme (GBE). This in turn results in accumulation of abnormal glycogen molecules that have longer outer chains and fewer branch points. GSD-IV manifests in a wide spectrum, with variable phenotypes depending on the degree and type of tissues in which this abnormal glycogen accumulates. Typically, GSD-IV presents with rapidly progressive liver cirrhosis and death in early childhood. However, there is a severe congenital neuromuscular variant of GSD-IV that has been reported in the literature, with fewer than 20 patient cases thus far. We report an unusual case of GSD-IV neuromuscular variant in a late preterm female infant who was born to non-consanguineous healthy parents with previously healthy children. Prenatally, our patient was found to have decreased fetal movement and polyhydramnios warranting an early delivery. Postnatally, she had severe hypotonia and respiratory failure, with no hepatic or cardiac involvement. Extensive metabolic and neurological workup revealed no abnormalities. However, molecular analysis by whole-exome sequencing revealed two pathogenic variants in the *GBE1* gene. Our patient was thus a compound heterozygote of the two pathogenic variants: one of these was inherited from the mother [p. L490WfsX5 (c.1468delC)], and the other pathogenic variant was a de novo change [p.E449X (c.1245G>T)]. As expected in GSD-IV, diffuse intracytoplasmic periodic acid-Schiff-positive, diastase-resistant inclusions were found in the cardiac myocytes, hepatocytes, and skeletal muscle fibers of our patient.

Introduction

Glycogen storage diseases (GSDs) are a group of rare inherited metabolic disorders caused by abnormal synthesis or breakdown of glycogen, leading to accumulation of abnormal quantity, quality, or both, of glycogen in the tissues. Glycogen is synthesized by the enzymes glycogen synthase and glycogen branching enzyme (GBE), which function in forming α-1,4 and α-1,6 glucose linkages, respectively (Tay et al. 2004). The α-1,6 branching in the glycogen molecule increases its solubility by decreasing the osmotic strength. Additionally, the action of glycogen phosphorylase on the branched structure of the glycogen molecule makes more glucose monomers available for metabolic needs. Accumulation of this abnormal glycogen molecule that has a long outer chain and poor solubility causes irreversible tissue and organ damage, especially in the liver and muscles.

There are multiple forms of GSDs, each with a predilection for a certain age group. GSD-IV (also called Andersen disease, amylopectinosis, or polyglucosan body disease) is a rare autosomal recessive disease, with an estimated incidence of 1 in every 760,000–960,000 births (Tang et al. 1994). It results from deficient GBE activity. Human GBE cDNA has been cloned and has a length of ~3 kb (Thon et al. 1993). The coding sequence contains

Communicated by: Terry G.J. Derks, MD, PhD

T. Sandhu (✉) · A. Makkar
Department of Neonatology, The Children's Hospital at OU Medical Center, Oklahoma City, OK, USA
e-mail: tavleen-sandhu@ouhsc.edu

M. Polan
Division of Human Genetics, The Children's Hospital at OU Medical Center, Oklahoma City, OK, USA

Z. Yu · R. Lu
Department of Pathology, The Children's Hospital at OU Medical Center, Oklahoma City, OK, USA

2,106 bp, encoding 702 amino acids. Human GBE protein is located on chromosome 3p (Thon et al. 1993). In the absence of GBE, an abnormal glycogen called polyglucosan is formed; it has fewer branching points and longer outer chains than normal glycogen (Tay et al. 2004). This polyglucosan accumulates in all tissues to various degrees and results in different manifestations of disease.

The more classic form of GSD-IV, originally described by Anderson in 1956, involves the liver, leading to progressive cirrhosis of the liver (Andersen 1956). However, there also exists a neuromuscular variant of GSD-IV. This variant is distinguished into four different groups categorized by the age of onset: perinatal, congenital, juvenile, and adult forms. To our knowledge, fewer than 20 cases of genetically characterized fatal congenital neuromuscular variant of GSD-IV have been reported in the literature thus far (Tay et al. 2004; Tang et al. 1994; Zellweger et al. 1972; Bao et al. 1996; Assereto et al. 2007; Bruno et al. 2004, 2007; Lamperti et al. 2009).

Case Report

We describe a female infant born at 36 weeks and 4 days of gestation by an urgent cesarean delivery for concerns of non-reassuring fetal testing, biophysical profile of 6, and marked polyhydramnios. Ultrasound immediately prior to delivery was significant for IUGR<5th percentile, small fetal stomach, and polyhydramnios with AFI of 39. These findings were concerning for tracheoesophageal fistula. The infant was delivered limp, with no respiratory effort and undetectable heart rate. The infant required extensive resuscitation, including intubation, chest compressions, and epinephrine in the delivery room. Apgar scores were 1, 1, 1, 2, 3, and 5 at 1, 5, 10, 15, 20, and 25 min of life. The infant was taken to the NICU, and a therapeutic hypothermia protocol was initiated based on the extensive resuscitation measures, initial gases, and seizures within first hour of life. On initial assessment, the infant's neurological status was Sarnat stage 3. The admission exam was consistent, with a birth weight of 2,230 g, head circumference of 33.5 cm, and length of 48 cm. There was no spontaneous eye opening or limb movements. The suck, gag, rooting, moro, and deep tendon reflexes were absent. There was no response to noxious stimuli. The infant's tone was flaccid. She had no dysmorphic features or arthrogryposis. Flexion creases were normal. There was no cardiac murmur or organomegaly.

On further history, mother is a 24-year-old woman with two prior healthy children. She reported a sudden 20-pound weight gain over the last three weeks and decreased fetal movements since ~6 months of gestation, which had been attributed to her class III obesity. She denied exposure to or use of any drugs, tobacco, or alcohol during pregnancy.

Both parents were reportedly healthy, had no significant family history of neuromuscular disorders, and denied consanguinity. The infant's exam remained unchanged over the course of the following weeks, other than for occasional movements of her finger and tongue. Initial echoencephalogram showed a structurally normal brain with no bleeds. Echocardiography showed a structurally normal heart, with signs of pulmonary hypertension on the initial day of life. Electroencephalogram was consistent with mild encephalopathy. Brain MRI and MR venogram showed no evidence of acute ischemia or sinus venous thrombosis. Extensive metabolic workup, including blood gases, blood glucose, serum amino acids, urine organic acids, ammonia, lactate, thyroid studies, acylcarnitine profile, gamma-glutamyltransferase, transaminases, aldolase, creatine kinase, and initial and repeat newborn screens, were all within normal limits. The sepsis workup done during hospital stay was negative. Additionally, the placental pathology was unremarkable. Single nucleotide polymorphism (SNP) array, whole-exome sequencing, and sequential analysis with deletion testing of the mitochondrial genome were performed.

The infant was noted to have hypercarbia when challenged with low ventilator settings and was thought to be ventilator-dependent. On day 29 of life, after extensive discussion with the family, the parents agreed to withdraw care because of the unfavorable prognosis. The patient was extubated and expired within minutes after the extubation. An unrestricted autopsy was performed immediately after death. At time of the autopsy, the baby weighed 2,590 g and the crown-heel length was 43 cm. There were no apparent dysmorphic features or evidence of congenital malformations. The most significant histological findings included diffuse intracytoplasmic, pale basophilic inclusions in the cardiac myocytes, hepatocytes, and skeletal muscle fibers [Fig. 1, upper panel (a–d)]. These inclusions were strongly positive for periodic acid-Schiff (PAS) staining [Fig. 1, middle panel (e–h)] and resistant to diastase digestion, i.e., positive for PAS-diastase staining [Fig. 1, lower panel (i–l)], which are consistent with indigestible abnormal polysaccharide material and support the diagnosis of type IV glycogen storage disease.

SNP array performed on the patient's peripheral blood did not reveal any clinically significant microdeletion or micro-duplication. Five small regions of homozygosity were identified, and the gene of interest was not a part of it. Subsequently, whole-exome sequencing further confirmed the diagnosis. The patient was noted to have two pathogenic variants in the *GBE1* gene, one resulting from a de novo change p.E449X (c.1345G>T) and the other inherited from the mother p.L490WfsX5 (c.1468delC). Pathogenic variants in *GBE1* gene are known to cause autosomal recessive GSD-IV. Clinical presentation, along with positive pathology findings suggestive of GSD-IV and

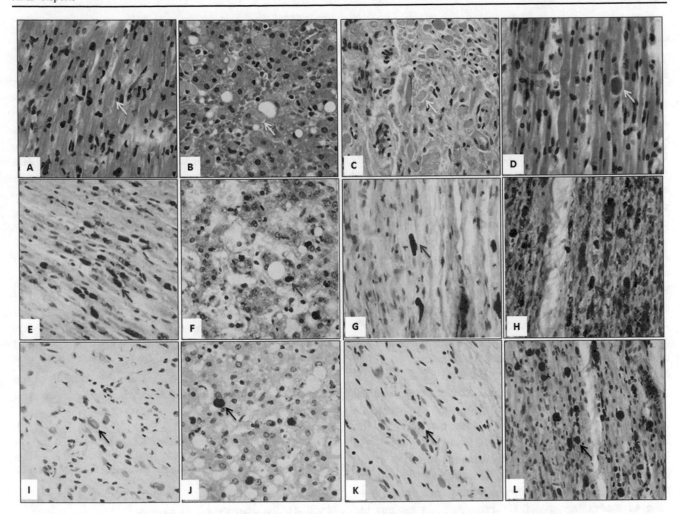

Fig. 1 Histopathological features of diffuse intracytoplasmic inclusions in the myocardial fibers (**a**, **e**, **i**), hepatocytes (**b**, **f**, **j**), intercostal skeletal muscle fibers (**c**, **g**, **k**), and thigh skeletal muscle fibers (**d**, **h**, **l**). Top panel (**a** through **d**): Tissues with hematoxylin and eosin staining demonstrate intracytoplasmic, pale basophilic inclusions (indicated by yellow arrows). Middle panel (**e** through **h**): Tissues with periodic acid-Schiff (PAS) staining show strong PAS-positive intracytoplasmic eosinophilic inclusions (indicated by blue arrows). Lower panel (**i** through **l**): tissues with PAS-diastase staining highlight PAS-positive diastases-resistant intracytoplasmic eosinophilic inclusions (indicated by black arrows)

molecular findings of two pathogenic variants of the *GBE1* gene, is consistent with most severe neonatal neuromuscular presentation of autosomal recessive GSD-IV.

Discussion

GSD-IV is a heterogeneous disorder that presents with marked clinical variability. The most classic form is the hepatic form that presents with hepatosplenomegaly and failure to thrive by 18 months of age, followed by progressive liver failure, and death by 5 years of age (Andersen 1956; Bao et al. 1996). The milder form involves nonprogressive hepatic dysfunction, which has little impact on life expectancy and does not necessitate liver transplantation (McConkie-Rosell et al. 1996). In addition to the more common hepatic form, there exists a neuromuscular variant,

which is further classified into four forms based on age at manifestation. The perinatal form of this variant presents with fetal akinesia, arthrogryposis, fetal hydrops, and death in the perinatal period (Alegria et al. 1999). The congenital form manifests with polyhydramnios, profound hypotonia, respiratory failure, and death in early infancy (Tay et al. 2004; Tang et al. 1994; Zellweger et al. 1972; Bao et al. 1996; Assereto et al. 2007; Bruno et al. 2004, 2007; Lamperti et al. 2009; McMaster et al. 1979). The juvenile form presents with hypotonia and/or cardiomyopathy (Bao et al. 1996; Reusche et al. 1992). Lastly, the adult-onset disease presents with diffuse central and peripheral nervous system dysfunction (Bruno et al. 1993).

Literature search yielded a handful of case reports on congenital GSD-IV, all with some variations in their clinical presentation. In 1972, Zellweger et al. reported

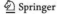

one of the earliest demonstrated GBE-deficient cases of infantile onset of GSD-IV with hypotonia (Zellweger et al. 1972). Tang et al. described a neonate with severe hypotonia and dilated cardiomyopathy without liver involvement, but amylopectin-like inclusions were found in hepatocytes, as seen in our patient (Tang et al. 1994). Tay et al. reported two unrelated patients with the congenital variant of GSD-IV, confirmed by pathogenic variants in the *GBE1* gene (Tay et al. 2004). Both pregnancies were complicated by polyhydramnios, and both neonates showed hypotonia and poor respiratory effort at birth. Autopsy results showed pale, atrophic skeletal muscles, and PAS-positive, diastase-resistant globules in the liver, heart, skeletal muscle, and neurons of the brain and spinal cord. Assereto et al. described two unrelated newborns who showed severe hypotonia at birth and died of cardiorespiratory failure at ages 4 and 12 weeks, respectively (Assereto et al. 2007). Both pregnancies were complicated by polyhydramnios and reduced fetal movements. *GBE1* activity in cultured fibroblasts was less than 5% in both cases. Molecular analysis identified a homozygous null mutation in the *2* gene in each patient.

Bruno et al., Burrow et al., and Fernandez et al. reported a total of four cases of non-lethal congenital hypotonia due to GSD-IV (Bruno et al. 2004; Burrow et al. 2006; Fernandez et al. 2010). All patients had significant delays in motor development, which plateaued at some point, leaving them wheelchair-bound. The degree of fine motor, language, and social impairments in these cases varied from none to moderately affected. These findings support the current theory of GSD-IV being a phenotypic spectrum with varying degrees of organ involvement, age of onset, and evolution of disease process, all dependent on the residual GBE activity (Fernandez et al. 2010). All cases of perinatal or neonatal death from GSD-IV have been associated with the near-complete absence of GBE activity (Assereto et al. 2007; Bruno et al. 2004, 2007).

We have reported here the clinical, pathological, and molecular data of an infant affected with GBE deficiency caused by de novo disease-causing one variant and another disease-causing variant inherited from the mother in the *GBE1* gene. Our patient's de novo p.E449X (c.1345G>T) variant in the *GBE1* gene is predicted to cause loss of normal protein function through either protein truncation or nonsense-mediated mRNA decay. This variant has not been previously reported as a pathogenic variant nor as a benign variant, but for our patient, it was interpreted as a pathogenic variant. The maternally inherited p.L490WfsX5 (c.1468delC) variant in the GBE1 gene has been reported previously in GSD-IV. This variant causes a frameshift starting with a codon Leucine 940, changes this amino acid to a tryptophan, and creates a premature stop codon at position 5 of the new reading frame.

Our patient demonstrated features of severe congenital GSD-IV, with profound hypotonia, polyhydramnios, respiratory failure, and no clinical liver or heart involvement. Diagnosis for our patient was made based on the accumulation of PAS-positive, diastase-resistant intracytoplasmic inclusions in hepatocytes, cardiac myocytes, and skeletal muscle fibers. In cases of autosomal recessive disorders, we normally expect both parents to be carriers of the disease-causing variants, but this was not the case for our patient. Only the mother of our patient was found to be a carrier for this variant; the second disease-causing variant happened as a new genetic change (de novo) in our patient. The risk for these parents to have another child affected with GSD-IV is minimal in this scenario.

The neuromuscular variant of GSD-IV is very rare. However, there is a strong possibility of underdiagnosis. The neuromuscular variant of GSD-IV should be considered one of the differential diagnoses in neonates with hypotonia and in pregnancies complicated with polyhydramnios, fetal hydrops, and reduced fetal movement of unknown etiology. The presence of PAS-positive and diastase-resistant inclusion bodies in the muscle is the hallmark for this disease, and gene sequencing is the gold standard for diagnosis.

Acknowledgment We thank Kathy Kyler for editorial support throughout writing process. We thank Drs. Henry Tran and Kar-Ming Fung for their assistant in sampling and examining the thigh muscular tissue.

Compliance with Ethics Guidelines

Tavleen Sandhu, Michelle Polan, Zhongxin Yu, Rufei Lu, and Abhishek Makkar declare that they have no conflicts of interest.

Tavleen Sandhu and Abhishek Makkar were the members of the primary medical team for the patient and were involved in planning, conduct, and reporting of the case. Michelle Polan, Zhongxin Yu, and Rufei Lu were part of the consultancy team and were involved in reporting of the case. Abhishek Makkar is the guarantor for this manuscript.

References

Alegria A, Martins E, Dias M, Cunha A, Cardoso ML, Maire I (1999) Glycogen storage disease type IV presenting as hydrops fetalis. J Inherit Metab Dis 22:330–332

Andersen DH (1956) Familial cirrhosis of the liver with storage of abnormal glycogen. Lab Invest 5:11–20

Assereto S, van Diggelen OP, Diogo L et al (2007) Null mutations and lethal congenital form of glycogen storage disease type IV. Biochem Biophys Res Commun 361:445–450

Bao Y, Kishnani P, Wu JY, Chen YT (1996) Hepatic and neuromuscular forms of glycogen storage disease type IV caused by mutations in the same glycogen-branching enzyme gene. J Clin Invest 97:941–948

Bruno C, Servidei S, Shanske S et al (1993) Glycogen branching enzyme deficiency in adult polyglucosan body disease. Ann Neurol 33:88–93

Bruno C, van Diggelen OP, Cassandrini D et al (2004) Clinical and genetic heterogeneity of branching enzyme deficiency (glycogenosis type IV). Neurology 63:1053–1058

Bruno C, Cassandrini D, Assereto S, Akman HO, Minetti C, Di Mauro S (2007) Neuromuscular forms of glycogen branching enzyme deficiency. Acta Myol 26:75–78

Burrow TA, Hopkin RJ, Bove KE et al (2006) Non-lethal congenital hypotonia due to glycogen storage disease type IV. Am J Med Genet A 140:878–882

Fernandez C, Halbert C, De Paula AM et al (2010) Non-lethal neonatal neuromuscular variant of glycogenosis type IV with novel GBE1 mutations. Muscle Nerve 41:269–271

Lamperti C, Salani S, Lucchiari S et al (2009) Neuropathological study of skeletal muscle, heart, liver, and brain in a neonatal form of glycogen storage disease type IV associated with a new mutation in GBE1 gene. J Inherit Metab Dis 32(Suppl 1): S161–S168

McConkie-Rosell A, Wilson C, Piccoli DA et al (1996) Clinical and laboratory findings in four patients with the non-progressive hepatic form of type IV glycogen storage disease. J Inherit Metab Dis 19:51–58

McMaster KR, Powers JM, Hennigar GR Jr, Wohltmann HJ, Farr GH Jr (1979) Nervous system involvement in type IV glycogenosis. Arch Pathol Lab Med 103:105–111

Reusche E, Aksu F, Goebel HH, Shin YS, Yokota T, Reichmann H (1992) A mild juvenile variant of type IV glycogenosis. Brain Dev 14:36–43

Tang TT, Segura AD, Chen YT et al (1994) Neonatal hypotonia and cardiomyopathy secondary to type IV glycogenosis. Acta Neuropathol 87:531–536

Tay SK, Akman HO, Chung WK et al (2004) Fatal infantile neuromuscular presentation of glycogen storage disease type IV. Neuromuscul Disord 14:253–260

Thon VJ, Khalil M, Cannon JF (1993) Isolation of human glycogen branching enzyme cDNAs by screening complementation in yeast. J Biol Chem 268:7509–7513

Zellweger H, Mueller S, Ionasescu V, Schochet SS, McCormick WF (1972) Glycogenosis. IV. A new cause of infantile hypotonia. J Pediatr 80:842–844

JIMD Reports
DOI 10.1007/8904_2018_136

RESEARCH REPORT

Acute and Chronic Management in an Atypical Case of Ethylmalonic Encephalopathy

**Thomas M. Kitzler · Indra R. Gupta ·
Bradley Osterman · Chantal Poulin · Yannis Trakadis ·
Paula J. Waters · Daniela C. Buhas**

Received: 01 March 2018 / Revised: 01 August 2018 / Accepted: 17 August 2018 / Published online: 23 October 2018
© Society for the Study of Inborn Errors of Metabolism (SSIEM) 2018

Abstract Ethylmalonic encephalopathy (EE) is caused by mutations in the *ETHE1* gene. ETHE1 is vital for the catabolism of hydrogen sulfide (H_2S). Patients with pathogenic mutations in *ETHE1* have markedly increased thiosulfate, which is a reliable index of H_2S levels. Accumulation of H_2S is thought to cause the characteristic metabolic derangement found in EE. Recently introduced treatment strategies in EE, such as combined use of metronidazole (MNZ) and N-acetylcysteine (NAC), are aimed at lowering chronic H_2S load. Experience with treatment strategies directed against acute episodes of metabolic decompensation (e.g., hemodialysis) is limited.

Communicated by: Ivo Barić, M.D., PhD, Professor of Pediatrics

Electronic supplementary material: The online version of this chapter (https://doi.org/10.1007/8904_2018_136) contains supplementary material, which is available to authorized users.

T. M. Kitzler (✉) · Y. Trakadis · D. C. Buhas
Department of Medical Genetics, McGill University Health Centre, Montreal, QC, Canada
e-mail: thomas.kitzler@mail.mcgill.ca

I. R. Gupta
Department of Pediatrics, Division of Nephrology, McGill University Health Centre, Montreal, QC, Canada

B. Osterman
Department of Pediatric Neurology, Centre Hospitalier de l'Université Laval (CHUL), Quebec City, QC, Canada

C. Poulin
Department of Pediatrics, Division of Neurology, McGill University Health Centre, Montreal, QC, Canada

P. J. Waters
Medical Genetics Service, Department of Pediatrics, University of Sherbrooke Hospital Centre (CHUS), Sherbrooke, QC, Canada

Here we present an unusually mild, molecularly confirmed, case of EE in a 19-year-old male on chronic treatment with MNZ and NAC. During an acute episode of metabolic decompensation, we employed continuous renal replacement therapy (CRRT) to regain metabolic control. On continuous treatment with NAC and MNZ during the months preceding the acute event, plasma thiosulfate levels ranged from 1.6 to 4 µg/mL (reference range up to 2 µg/mL) and had a mean value of 2.5 µg/mL. During the acute decompensation, thiosulfate levels were 6.7 µg/mL, with hyperlactatemia and perturbed organic acid, acylglycine, and acylcarnitine profiles. CRRT decreased thiosulfate within 24 h to 1.4 µg/mL. Following discontinuation of CRRT, mean thiosulfate levels were 3.2 µg/mL (range, 2.4–3.7 µg/mL) accompanied by clinical improvement with metabolic stabilization of blood gas, acylcarnitine, organic acid, and acylglycine profiles. In conclusion, CRRT may help to regain metabolic control in patients with EE who have an acute metabolic decompensation on chronic treatment with NAC and MNZ.

Introduction

Ethylmalonic encephalopathy (EE; OMIM #602473) is generally considered a rare autosomal recessive neurometabolic disorder of infancy but presents with wide clinical heterogeneity. It is clinically characterized by neurodevelopmental delay and regression, prominent pyramidal and extrapyramidal signs, recurrent petechiae, orthostatic acrocyanosis, and chronic diarrhea (Drousiotou et al. 2011). It was first described by Burlina et al. in 1991, but it was not until 2004 that Tiranti et al. mapped its genomic locus to the *ETHE1* gene (OMIM #608451) on chromosome 19q13 (Burlina et al. 1991; Tiranti et al. 2004). The *ETHE1* gene encodes a 30-kDa polypeptide (ETHE1), which is a non-heme, iron-dependent, mitochondrial matrix sulfur dioxygenase that is involved in the catabolism of hydrogen sulfide (H_2S). It catalyzes the oxidation of glutathione persulfide (GSSH) to give glutathione and persulfite (Kabil and Banerjee 2012; Pettinati et al. 2015).

$$GSSH + O_2 + H_2O \xrightarrow{hETHE1} GSH + SO_3^{2-} + 2H^+$$

This reaction is a vital part of the H_2S catabolic pathway, as it generates the glutathione (GSH) that is needed for the extraction of sulfur atoms of the intermediately produced thiosulfate (Hildebrandt and Grieshaber 2008; Jackson et al. 2012).

Hydrogen sulfide is a colorless, water-soluble gasotransmitter with physiologic roles in CNS signaling, heart rate regulation, blood pressure regulation, and inflammation (Kimura and Kimura 2004; Nagai et al. 2004; Qingyou et al. 2004; Whiteman et al. 2004; Xu et al. 2008; Bucci et al. 2010; Elsey et al. 2010). In mammals, H_2S can be endogenously produced from L-cysteine taken up by diet or synthesized via trans-sulfuration of serine by L-methionine, but most of the H_2S load stems from intestinal anaerobes (Viscomi et al. 2010; Di Meo et al. 2015). Under steady-state conditions, tissue concentrations of H_2S are generally in the low nanomolar range, but patients harboring biallelic pathogenic mutations in *ETHE1* were found to have markedly elevated levels of thiosulfate, which can be used as a stable and readily measurable index of H_2S levels (Viscomi et al. 2010). The accumulated H_2S inhibits short-chain acyl CoA dehydrogenase (SCAD) and cytochrome c oxidase (COX) activities, causing the characteristic, but far from specific, biochemical changes observed in patients with EE, namely, *ethylmalonic acid (EMA) aciduria*, sometimes with mild elevations of short-chain acylglycines also detected in the urine organic acid profile (*ethylmalonic acid, methylsuccinic acid, isobutyrylglycine,* and *iso-valerylglycine*), increased levels of plasma *C4-* and *C5-acylcarnitines*, and elevated *plasma lactate* (Tiranti et al. 2009). The ensuing metabolic derangement is thought to cause damages to the intestinal mucosa and the endothelia and lead to alterations of the blood vessel tone, thereby resulting in the main clinical features of EE (e.g., chronic hemorrhagic and/or mucoid diarrhea, petechial purpura with edematous acrocyanosis, and progressive neurological failure with pyramidal signs).

Treatment

There are several reports in the literature of patients that have been diagnosed with EE through newborn screening, during routine medical referral, or through a known family history, which contributed to our understanding of chronic management of this disease (Grosso et al. 2002; McGowan et al. 2004; Zafeiriou et al. 2007; Mineri et al. 2008; Pigeon et al. 2009; Dionisi-Vici et al. 2016; Tavasoli et al. 2017; Boyer et al. 2018). This has led to the introduction of new treatment strategies, such as the combined use of antibiotics and N-acetylcysteine (NAC), which is aimed at lowering the chronic H_2S load (Viscomi et al. 2010). Metronidazole (MNZ) is a commonly used bactericidal nitroimidazole that is broadly active against aerobic and anaerobic bacterial species (Perencevich and Burakoff 2006). N-acetylcysteine, on the other hand, is a cell-permeable precursor of GSH, which is needed as an acceptor of sulfur atoms in H_2S catabolism (Atkuri et al. 2007). Notably, a recent report by Boyer et al. suggests that a diet restricted in sulfur-containing amino acids, in addition to medical treatment, results in further improvement in clinical outcomes and biochemical markers in patients with EE identified on newborn screening (Boyer et al. 2018). Despite these advances, our knowledge of chronic management of EE remains scant, due to the rarity of the disease and the fact that many cases of EE described in the literature presented within the first year of life in context of an acute metabolic decompensation with an almost invariably lethal outcome.

Here we describe our experience with the use of continuous renal replacement therapy (CRRT) to lower plasma sulfide levels in an unusually mild clinical course of EE in a 19-year-old male, who nonetheless presented with an acute metabolic decompensation, despite chronic treatment with antibiotics and NAC. To the best of our knowledge, the use of continuous veno-venous hemodialysis was reported only once before in a case of EE to remove EE-associated metabolites during liver transplant surgery (Dionisi-Vici et al. 2016).

Case Report

Our patient is a 19-year-old man with an atypical mild form of EE. He was initially seen at the department of Medical Genetics at 10 years of age because of long-standing spastic paraplegia, dysarthria, and Arnold-Chiari malformation type I of unclear etiology. He was also regularly followed at the department of Pediatric Neurology for treatment of his spastic paraplegia with a baclofen pump. He had no history of diarrhea or acrocyanosis. The clinical features are summarized in Table 1. His parents are a non-consanguineous couple from Serbia, and he has an older healthy brother.

First Hospitalization

At 16 years of age, he was admitted to the pediatric ICU for generalized spasticity and trismus in the context of an upper respiratory tract infection. Metabolic work-up revealed

Table 1 Summary of clinical features

Clinical features reported in EE	Absent or present (− or +)
Failure to thrive	−
Retinal lesions with tortuous vessels	n/a
Orthostatic acrocyanosis	−
Chronic diarrhea	−
Petechiae	−
Coma/encephalopathy	During metabolic decompensation
Developmental regression	−
Developmental delay	+
Intellectual disability	+
Pyramidal symptoms	+
Ataxia	+
Hypotonia	−
Seizures	During metabolic decompensation
Hyperintense lesions in the basal ganglia on MRI	+
Other clinical features not reported in EE	
Trismus	During first hospitalization

n/a not assessed

elevated C4-carnitine on plasma acylcarnitine profile, although without substantial elevation of C5-carnitine, and moderately elevated EMA on urine organic acid profile on three consecutive measurements (72, 29, and 42 mmol/mol creatinine, reference range <11) along with slightly elevated methylsuccinic acid levels and variable slight elevations of short-chain acylglycines. Plasma lactate was within the normal range on multiple samples. The rest of the metabolic work-up was unremarkable. An MRI of the brain showed bilateral and symmetric increased T2 signaling in the basal ganglia and cerebellum (Fig. 1a, b). Magnetic resonance spectroscopy (MRS) of the basal ganglia demonstrated a corresponding high lactate peak not shown. Sanger sequencing of the *ETHE1* gene identified a homozygous missense variant (c.79C>A; p. Gln27Lys) for which both parents were carriers. Interestingly, the same mutation (in heterozygous status with another known pathogenic variant) was described in two sisters with EE, also coming from former Yugoslavia (Pigeon et al. 2009). The acute management during this admission was supportive with IV fluids, dextrose, and carnitine, and, based on his biochemical profile, MNZ and NAC were added for treatment of suspected EE. After discharge and upon molecular confirmation, chronic treatment with MNZ 500 mg tid (1 week on, 1 week off) and NAC at 100 mg/kg/day divided tid was initiated, and plasma thiosulfate levels were measured regularly to assess metabolic control. Over the next 12 months, his plasma

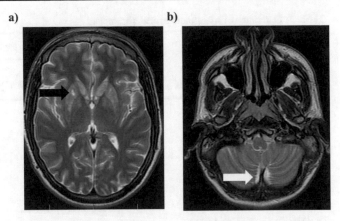

Fig. 1 MRI brain images during the first hospitalization. (**a**) T2-weighted image demonstrating signal hyperintensity at the level of the basal ganglia (black arrow). (**b**) T2-weighted image demonstrating signal hyperintensity at the level of the cerebellum (white arrow)

thiosulfate levels ranged from 1.6 to 4 μg/mL (reference <2 μg/mL), and he demonstrated significant improvement in mobility and speech.

Second Hospitalization with Acute Metabolic Decompensation

At 17 years of age, the patient was admitted to the pediatric psychiatric ward for an episode of suicidal ideation. During the admission, he developed a severe metabolic decompensation with encephalopathy, new-onset focal seizures, fever, and high lactate with no identifiable trigger and, while on sufficient caloric intake, required intubation and admission to intensive care. His plasma thiosulfate levels increased from 2.5 to 6.7 μg/mL, and plasma lactate levels were as high as 14.8 mmol/L (reference range 0.6–2.4). Quantitative urine acylglycine profile analysis (Bherer et al. 2015) showed elevations of several C4, C5, and other species, with butyrylglycine (C4) at 16.95 mmol/mol creatinine (reference range, 0.01–0.15 mmol/mol creatinine) being the most markedly elevated during the acute episode. Table 2 summarizes laboratory investigations pre, post, and during the acute events, while Supplementary Table 1 summarizes results for EMA, other organic acids, and acylglycine profile from multiple samples collected during the acute episodes and on other occasions. Plasma acylcarnitine profiling persistently showed C4-carnitine elevation in all samples. Multiple other acylcarnitines were elevated only at the time of this acute episode, although notably C5-carnitine was never substantially elevated (see Table 2). Figure 2 summarizes the MRI images taken during this episode, which demonstrated new evidence of acute and chronic brain injury (Fig. 2a–c). While trying to identify the underlying trigger of this acute episode, it was

Table 2 Summary of main biochemical parameters

Clinical status	Lactate (plasma) (0.6–2.2)[a]	Thiosulfate (plasma) <2[b]	Plasma acylcarnitines[c] C4 (0.06–0.44)	C5 (0.03–0.24)	Urine organic acids[d] and acylglycines[e] EMA[f] (<11)	Isobutyryl (0.08–1.59)	Butyryl (0.01–0.15)	Isovaleryl (0.14–2.98)
First hospitalization	1	–	*2.4*	*0.47*	72	–	–	–
First hospitalization	1.4	–	*6.71*	*0.92*	–	–	–	–
Stable interim period	2.0	1.5	*1.02*	0.17	–	–	–	–
DOD[g] – *12 days*	1.7	1.6	–	–	–	–	–	–
DOD1[g,h]	*7.7*	*3.3*	*1.14*	0.19	*100*	*7.48*	*16.95*	*8.32*
DOD2[g,h]	*10.6*	*5.4*	–	–	–	–	–	–
DOD3[g,h]	*14.3*	*6.7*	–	–	–	–	–	–
DOD4[g,h,i]	*14.8*	–	–	–	–	–	–	–
DOD5[g,h,i]	*12.9*	1.4	–	–	–	–	–	–
DOD6[g,h,i]	*9.7*	*2.7*	*0.71*	0.19	*13*	0.90	*0.85*	2.65
DOD7[g,h]	*5.9*	*3.7*	*0.80*	0.18	*18*	–	–	–
DOD8[g,h]	*3.6*	*2.4*	*1.14*	0.20	*20*	–	–	–
DOD9	*2.3*	–	–	–	–	–	–	–
Stable	<2.2	*3.6*	–	–	–	–	–	–

[a] Lactate – highest day level is indicated. Concentrations expressed in mmol/L; reference values shown in parentheses; *italic* values are above reference range

[b] Thiosulfate, analysis by ion chromatography (NMS labs, USA). Concentrations expressed in mcg/mL; reference values shown; *italic* values are above reference range

[c] Acylcarnitines. Concentrations expressed in umol/L; reference values shown in parentheses; *italic* values are above reference range

[d] Urine organic acids. Concentrations expressed in mmol/mol creatinine; reference values shown in parentheses; *italic* values are above reference range

[e] Urine acylglycines. Concentrations expressed in mmol/mol creatinine; reference values shown in parentheses; *italic* values are above reference range

[f] *EMA* ethylmalonic acid

[g] *DOD* day of decompensation

[h] Received IV carnitine

[i] Received CRRT

noted that the subcutaneous baclofen pump was empty, and concerns were raised about the possibility of a baclofen intoxication. Notably, continuous EEG recordings showed moderate to severe disturbance of cerebral activity with patterns suggestive of baclofen toxicity (e.g., triphasic waves, frontal intermittent rhythmic delta activity alternating with faster rhythms in the theta and alpha range) (Sutter et al. 2018). This could not be confirmed by measurement of CSF baclofen levels, which were undetectable. Notably, the CSF sample was drawn only on day 5 of the acute event, 2 days after initiation of CRRT, due to the patient's clinical instability.

Despite intensive supportive management (IV fluids, dextrose, MNZ, NAC, carnitine, and appropriate caloric intake) over 3 days, there was worsening of the patient's clinical and metabolic state, reflected by increasing lactate levels. Although his renal function remained intact (serum creatinine 63 mmol/L with good urine output), additional treatment with CRRT was initiated on day 4 and continued

for 96 h in the form of continuous venovenous hemodiafiltration (CVVHDF). The CVVHDF prescription included a blood flow of 200 mL/min, dialysate flow of 1.2 L/h, and replacement flow of 1.2 L/h. This rapidly lowered thiosulfate, lactate, and other biochemical parameters to baseline levels and allowed us to regain metabolic control (Fig. 3 and Supplementary Table 1). The improved metabolic state was accompanied by a reversal of the encephalopathy and restoration of consciousness. Over the following weeks, the patient continued his recovery and could regain much of his functionality.

Discussion

To this day, more than 80 patients have received a molecular diagnosis of EE (Tiranti et al. 2004, 2006; Mineri et al. 2008; Drousiotou et al. 2011; Tiranti and Zeviani 2013). The natural history of the disease was thought to be invariably fatal with onset in the first

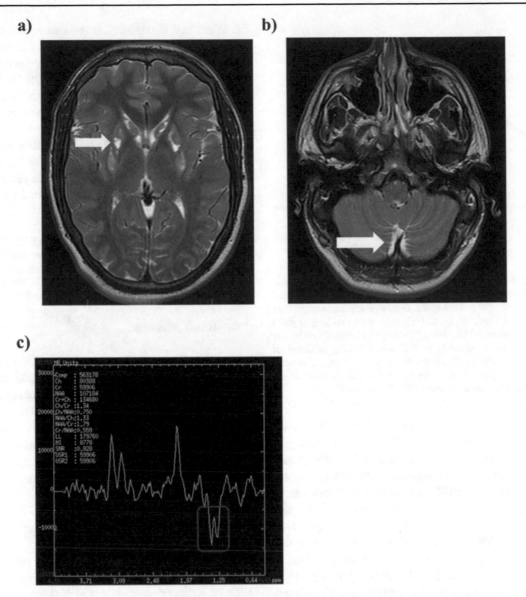

Fig. 2 MRI brain images during the second episode of acute metabolic decompensation. (**a**) T2-weighted images demonstrated interval atrophy and central necrosis of the known basal ganglia abnormality with a new area of hyperintensity (white arrow) and corresponding diffusion restriction along the posterior putamina. (**b**) At the level of the cerebellum, there was abnormal symmetric hyperintensity in the dentate nuclei and the inferior cerebellar subcortical white matter (white arrow). (**c**) Multivoxel MRS demonstrated an inverted lactate peak in the basal ganglia and centrum semiovale at 1.3 ppm. The inverted lactate peak on MRS corresponds to an elevated tissue lactate. At 1.3 ppm, lactate resonates with a characteristic double peak at long echo times but is superimposed on the lipid band. By using an intermediate echo time of 135–145 ms, the lactate peak will be inverted, allowing it to be distinguished

2–4 months of life, which is followed by progressive clinical deterioration with psychomotor regression and complete absence of neurological improvement. However, the two sisters (monochorionic twins) reported by Pigeon et al., harboring one of the same mutations as our patient, had a milder disease course suggesting a genotype-phenotype correlation (Pigeon et al. 2009). Like our patient, both sisters lacked the characteristic features of EE, such as petechiae, orthostatic acrocyanosis, or chronic diarrhea. Of note, despite them being monochorionic twins, their clinical courses differed markedly; one had an episode of coma at 3 years of age, had spastic quadriparesis at 10 years of age, and could not speak, while the other sister had pyramidal symptoms mostly limited to the lower extremities and was able to speak two languages. As mentioned by Pigeon et al., this observation highlights the marked clinical heterogeneity displayed in EE. Insight into the biochemical nature of EE has led to the advent of new treatment strategies aimed at lowering the chronic H_2S load (e.g., MNZ and NAC). Recently, Dionisi-Vici et al. convincingly reported the successful use of liver transplantation as an effective therapeutic approach in reverting the natural course of an

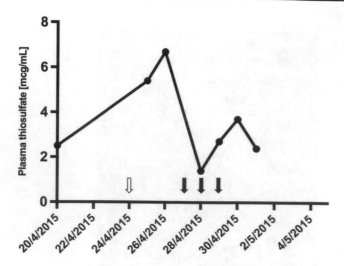

Fig. 3 Plasma thiosulfate levels during the second episode of acute metabolic decompensation. On continuous treatment with NAC and MNZ during the months preceding the acute event, plasma thiosulfate levels ranged from 1.6 to 4 μg/mL (reference range up to 2 μg/mL) and had a mean value of 2.5 μg/mL. During the acute decompensation, thiosulfate levels increased to 6.7 μg/mL. After initiation of CRRT over 3 days, plasma thiosulfate levels rapidly returned to near-normal values. The white arrow indicates the onset of the acute event. Black arrows indicate the days when CRRT was given

otherwise fatal neurological disease (Dionisi-Vici et al. 2016). However, experience with treatment strategies directed against acute episodes of metabolic decompensation (e.g., hemodialysis) in patients with milder disease forms, who may not qualify for liver transplantation, is limited, except for a recent report of the use of IV NAC in a patient with an acute episode of EE in the context of meningococcemia (Kilic et al. 2017). Here we share our experience with an unusually mild clinical course of EE in a 19-year-old male, who presented with two acute episodes, one being an acute metabolic decompensation. His second episode was characterized by increasingly elevated lactate levels and metabolic deterioration, as reflected by levels of plasma thiosulfate and other biochemical parameters, despite intensive supportive management. To regain control of his metabolic state, we successfully employed CRRT to lower plasma sulfide levels. Given the small size of thiosulfate (112 D), these anions are readily removed by convection from hemofiltration and/or diffusion from dialysis; therefore, our patient received both modalities delivered as CVVHDF. Importantly, CRRT removes NAC but has no appreciable effect on the removal of MNZ (Hernandez et al. 2015; Roberts et al. 2015). It is suggested that the dose of intravenous NAC should be doubled during dialytic therapies. Notably, when we measured baclofen in CSF, levels were undetectable. It is important to point out that the CSF sample could only be obtained on day 5 of the acute episode. Around 70–80% of baclofen is excreted in

the urine, and about 15% is metabolized in the liver. The elimination half-life is about 5 h in CSF but has been reported to increase up to 35 h in overdose (Meulendijks et al. 2015). However, given that CRRT is known to improve baclofen clearance, it is conceivable that, after 5 days, most of the baclofen may have been eliminated (Roberts et al. 2015).

In conclusion, CRRT may help to regain metabolic control in patients with milder courses of EE with an acute metabolic decompensation who are on chronic treatment with NAC and MNZ and fail to respond to conventional supportive measures.

Acknowledgments We would like to thank the patient and his family for giving us permission to publish this case report. We also thank Patrick Bherer (of the CHUS biochemical genetics laboratory) for analysis of urine acylglycine profiles and Dr. Massimo Zeviani for his advice during the second acute decompensation.

Take-Home Message

By reading this case report on a patient with an unusually mild form of ethylmalonic encephalopathy (EE), readers will learn about the acute and chronic management of this rare condition and about the importance of keeping metabolic causes, such as EE, in mind in patients presenting with a purely neurological phenotype. Finally, our report illustrates the importance of identifying all possible triggers of a metabolic decompensation in patients with inborn errors of metabolism.

Author Contributions

TMK: Data analysis and interpretation and planning and drafting most of the article.
IRG: Article contribution and revision.
BO: Article contribution and revision.
CP: Article contribution and revision.
YT: Data analysis and interpretation and article contribution and revision.
PJW: Data analysis and interpretation and article contribution and revision.
DCB: Data analysis and interpretation and planning and drafting of article.

Competing Interests

The authors have no competing interests to declare.

Funding

This work has not received any funding.

Patient Consent

The patient and his parents provided informed consent for publication of this case report.

Ethical Standards

The authors declare that the experiments comply with the current laws of Canada, the country in which they were performed.

References

Atkuri KR, Mantovani JJ, Herzenberg LA, Herzenberg LA (2007) N-Acetylcysteine – a safe antidote for cysteine/glutathione deficiency. Curr Opin Pharmacol 7:355–359

Bherer P, Cyr D, Buhas D, Al-Hertani W, Maranda B, Waters PJ (2015) Acylglycine profiling: a new liquid chromatography-tandem mass spectrometry (LC-MS/MS) method, applied to disorders of organic acid, fatty acid, and ketone metabolism. J Inherit Metab Dis 38:S35–S378

Boyer M, Sowa M, Di Meo I et al (2018) Response to medical and a novel dietary treatment in newborn screen identified patients with ethylmalonic encephalopathy. Mol Genet Metab 124:57–63

Bucci M, Papapetropoulos A, Vellecco V et al (2010) Hydrogen sulfide is an endogenous inhibitor of phosphodiesterase activity. Arterioscler Thromb Vasc Biol 30:1998–2004

Burlina A, Zacchello F, Dionisi-Vici C et al (1991) New clinical phenotype of branched-chain acyl-CoA oxidation defect. Lancet 338:1522–1523

Di Meo I, Lamperti C, Tiranti V (2015) Mitochondrial diseases caused by toxic compound accumulation: from etiopathology to therapeutic approaches. EMBO Mol Med 7:1257–1266

Dionisi-Vici C, Diodato D, Torre G et al (2016) Liver transplant in cthylmalonic encephalopathy: a new treatment for an otherwise fatal disease. Brain 139:1045–1051

Drousiotou A, DiMeo I, Mineri R, Georgiou T, Stylianidou G, Tiranti V (2011) Ethylmalonic encephalopathy: application of improved biochemical and molecular diagnostic approaches. Clin Genet 79:385–390

Elsey DJ, Fowkes RC, Baxter GF (2010) Regulation of cardiovascular cell function by hydrogen sulfide (H(2)S). Cell Biochem Funct 28:95–106

Grosso S, Mostardini R, Farnetani MA et al (2002) Ethylmalonic encephalopathy: further clinical and neuroradiological characterization. J Neurol 249:1446–1450

Hernandez SH, Howland M, Schiano TD, Hoffman RS (2015) The pharmacokinetics and extracorporeal removal of N-acetylcysteine during renal replacement therapies. Clin Toxicol (Phila) 53:941–949

Hildebrandt TM, Grieshaber MK (2008) Three enzymatic activities catalyze the oxidation of sulfide to thiosulfate in mammalian and invertebrate mitochondria. FEBS J 275:3352–3361

Jackson MR, Melideo SL, Jorns MS (2012) Human sulfide:quinone oxidoreductase catalyzes the first step in hydrogen sulfide metabolism and produces a sulfane sulfur metabolite. Biochemistry 51:6804–6815

Kabil O, Banerjee R (2012) Characterization of patient mutations in human persulfide dioxygenase (ETHE1) involved in H2S catabolism. J Biol Chem 287:44561–44567

Kilic M, Dedeoglu O, Gocmen R, Kesici S, Yuksel D (2017) Successful treatment of a patient with ethylmalonic encephalopathy by intravenous N-acetylcysteine. Metab Brain Dis 32:293–296

Kimura Y, Kimura H (2004) Hydrogen sulfide protects neurons from oxidative stress. FASEB J 18:1165–1167

McGowan KA, Nyhan WL, Barshop BA et al (2004) The role of methionine in ethylmalonic encephalopathy with petechiae. Arch Neurol 61:570–574

Meulendijks D, Khan S, Koks CH, Huitema AD, Schellens JH, Beijnen JH (2015) Baclofen overdose treated with continuous venovenous hemofiltration. Eur J Clin Pharmacol 71:357–361

Mineri R, Rimoldi M, Burlina AB et al (2008) Identification of new mutations in the ETHE1 gene in a cohort of 14 patients presenting with ethylmalonic encephalopathy. J Med Genet 45:473–478

Nagai Y, Tsugane M, Oka J, Kimura H (2004) Hydrogen sulfide induces calcium waves in astrocytes. FASEB J 18:557–559

Perencevich M, Burakoff R (2006) Use of antibiotics in the treatment of inflammatory bowel disease. Inflamm Bowel Dis 12:651–664

Pettinati I, Brem J, McDonough MA, Schofield CJ (2015) Crystal structure of human persulfide dioxygenase: structural basis of ethylmalonic encephalopathy. Hum Mol Genet 24:2458–2469

Pigeon N, Campeau PM, Cyr D, Lemieux B, Clarke JT (2009) Clinical heterogeneity in ethylmalonic encephalopathy. J Child Neurol 24:991–996

Qingyou Z, Junbao D, Weijin Z, Hui Y, Chaoshu T, Chunyu Z (2004) Impact of hydrogen sulfide on carbon monoxide/heme oxygenase pathway in the pathogenesis of hypoxic pulmonary hypertension. Biochem Biophys Res Commun 317:30–37

Roberts JK, Westphal S, Sparks MA (2015) Iatrogenic baclofen neurotoxicity in ESRD: recognition and management. Semin Dial 28:525–529

Sutter R, Pang T, Kaplan PW (2018) Metabolic, toxic, and epileptic encephalopathies. Wolters Kluwer, Alphen aan den Rijn

Tavasoli AR, Rostami P, Ashrafi MR, Karimzadeh P (2017) Neurological and vascular manifestations of ethylmalonic encephalopathy. Iran J Child Neurol 11:57–60

Tiranti V, Zeviani M (2013) Altered sulfide (H(2)S) metabolism in ethylmalonic encephalopathy. Cold Spring Harb Perspect Biol 5: a011437

Tiranti V, D'Adamo P, Briem E et al (2004) Ethylmalonic encephalopathy is caused by mutations in ETHE1, a gene encoding a mitochondrial matrix protein. Am J Hum Genet 74:239–252

Tiranti V, Briem E, Lamantea E et al (2006) ETHE1 mutations are specific to ethylmalonic encephalopathy. J Med Genet 43:340–346

Tiranti V, Viscomi C, Hildebrandt T et al (2009) Loss of ETHE1, a mitochondrial dioxygenase, causes fatal sulfide toxicity in ethylmalonic encephalopathy. Nat Med 15:200–205

Viscomi C, Burlina AB, Dweikat I et al (2010) Combined treatment with oral metronidazole and N-acetylcysteine is effective in ethylmalonic encephalopathy. Nat Med 16:869–871

Whiteman M, Armstrong JS, Chu SH et al (2004) The novel neuromodulator hydrogen sulfide: an endogenous peroxynitrite 'scavenger'? J Neurochem 90:765–768

Xu M, Wu YM, Li Q, Wang X, He RR (2008) Electrophysiological effects of hydrogen sulfide on pacemaker cells in sinoatrial nodes of rabbits. Sheng Li Xue Bao 60:175–180

Zafeiriou DI, Augoustides-Savvopoulou P, Haas D et al (2007) Ethylmalonic encephalopathy: clinical and biochemical observations. Neuropediatrics 38:78–82

JIMD Reports
DOI 10.1007/8904_2018_138

Dihydropyrimidine Dehydrogenase Deficiency: Homozygosity for an Extremely Rare Variant in *DPYD* due to Uniparental Isodisomy of Chromosome 1

André B. P. van Kuilenburg · Judith Meijer · Rutger Meinsma · Belén Pérez-Dueñas · Marielle Alders · Zahurul A. Bhuiyan · Rafael Artuch · Raoul C. M. Hennekam

Received: 23 July 2018 / Revised: 17 August 2018 / Accepted: 20 August 2018 / Published online: 23 October 2018
© Society for the Study of Inborn Errors of Metabolism (SSIEM) 2018

Abstract Dihydropyrimidine dehydrogenase (DPD) deficiency is a rare autosomal recessive disorder of the pyrimidine degradation pathway and can lead to intellectual disability, motor retardation, and seizures. Genetic variations in *DPYD* have also emerged as predictive risk factors for severe toxicity in cancer patients treated with fluoropyrimidines. We recently observed a child born to nonconsanguineous parents, who demonstrated seizures, cognitive impairment, language delay, and MRI abnormalities and was found to have marked thymine-uraciluria. No residual DPD activity could be detected in peripheral blood mononuclear cells. Molecular analysis showed that the child was homozygous for the very rare c.257C > T (p. Pro86Leu) variant in *DPYD*. Functional analysis of the recombinantly expressed DPD mutant showed that the DPD mutant carrying the p.Pro86Leu did not possess any residual DPD activity. Carrier testing in parents revealed that the father was heterozygous for the variant but unexpectedly the mother did not carry the variant. Microsatellite repeat testing with markers covering chromosome 1 showed that the DPD deficiency in the child is due to paternal uniparental isodisomy. Our report thus extends the genetic spectrum underlying *DPYD* deficiency.

Introduction

Dihydropyrimidine dehydrogenase (DPD) is the initial and rate-limiting enzyme of the pyrimidine degradation pathway, catalyzing the reduction of uracil and thymine to 5,6-dihydrouracil and 5,6-dihydrothymine, respectively. In patients with a complete DPD deficiency (MIM 274270), a considerable variation in the clinical presentation has been observed ranging from severely (neurologically) affected to symptomless. Therefore, a DPD deficiency is probably a necessary, but not a sole prerequisite for the onset of a clinical phenotype (Fleger et al. 2017; van Kuilenburg et al. 1999). Delayed cognitive and motor development and convulsive disorders are relatively frequent manifestations, whereas growth retardation, microcephaly, dysmorphia, autism, hypotonia, and ocular abnormalities are less frequently observed (Chen et al. 2014; Enns et al. 2004; van Kuilenburg et al. 1999, 2002a, 2009). In addition, patients with a DPD deficiency have a strongly reduced capacity to degrade the widely used chemotherapeutic drug 5-fluorouracil and, therefore, an increased likelihood of suffering from severe and sometimes fatal multi-organ toxicity (Johnson and Diasio 2001; van Kuilenburg 2004).

Communicated by: Jörn Oliver Sass

A. B. P. van Kuilenburg (✉) · J. Meijer · R. Meinsma · M. Alders · R. C. M. Hennekam
Amsterdam UMC, University of Amsterdam, Departments of Clinical Chemistry, Genetics and Pediatrics, Amsterdam Gastroenterology & Metabolism, Amsterdam, The Netherlands
e-mail: a.b.vankuilenburg@amc.uva.nl

B. Pérez-Dueñas · R. Artuch
Departments of Neuropediatrics and Clinical Biochemistry, Institut de Recerca Sant Joan de Déu, CIBERER-ISCIII, Barcelona, Spain

B. Pérez-Dueñas
Vall d'Hebron Research Institute (VHIR), Universitat Autònoma de Barcelona, Barcelona, Spain

Z. A. Bhuiyan
Service de Médecine Génétique, Laboratoires de Médecine Génétique, Centre Hospitalier Universitaire Vaudois, Lausanne, Switzerland

DPYD is present as a single copy gene on chromosome 1p21.3 and consists of 23 exons (Wei et al. 1998). A large number of variants have been described in *DPYD* including large genomic deletions and amplifications (van Kuilenburg et al. 2009). The identification of novel disease-causing genomic aberrations is important to allow analysis of genotype-phenotype relationships in DPD-deficient patients and screening of cancer patients at risk. Our study identified a novel genetic mechanism underlying DPD deficiency, and we present the first patient with a complete DPD deficiency due to paternal uniparental isodisomy of chromosome 1.

Materials and Methods

Sequence analysis of *DPYD*, including analysis of intragenic rearrangements, was carried out essentially as described before (van Kuilenburg et al. 2017). Analysis of pyrimidine metabolites was performed using reversed-phase HPLC combined with electrospray tandem-mass spectrometry (van Lenthe et al. 2000). Functional expression of a *DPYD* mutation in mammalian HEK293 Flp-In cells and subsequent analysis of recombinantly expressed DPD protein levels and DPD activity were performed as described before (van Kuilenburg et al. 2017).

Twenty six microsatellite repeat markers spreading over the full length of chromosome 1 were used for haplotype analysis. These included 21 markers from ABI-Prism Linkage Mapping Set MD panels 1 and 2 (PE Biosystems, Foster City, CA, USA) and 5 additional markers: D1S2775, D1S2719, D1S2793, D1S415, and D1S2753 (NCBI, UniSTS). After PCR, the amplified fragments were separated using the ABI Prism 377 automatic DNA sequencer (PE Biosystems, Foster City, CA, USA), and the length of the fragments was analyzed with GeneMapper software (PE Biosystems, Foster City, CA, USA).

Results

Case Report

The female patient was the first child of non-consanguineous Portuguese parents. Developmental delay was noticed during the second year of life: she walked unassisted at the age of 20 months and showed language delay. At the age of 3 years, she started to have seizures. Despite treatment with valproic acid and carbamazepine, she continued to have seizures every few weeks to months. A neuropsychological study at 5 years and 8 months using the McCarthy Scales of Children's Abilities (MSCA) showed significantly reduced scores [verbal, 22; perceptual performance, 22; quantitative, 22; memory, 25; motor, 24 (controls: mean ± standard deviation 50 ± 10); and general cognitive index, 50

(controls: mean ± standard deviation 100 ± 15)]. Neurological examination at the age of 7 years revealed a non-dysmorphic child with normal growth and head circumference and poor fine and gross motor coordination. She was socially engaging and showed cognitive impairment and language delay. Magnetic resonance imaging (MRI) demonstrated symmetrically enlarged lateral ventricles and a thin corpus callosum. Cerebral white matter signal was normal. EEG showed generalized slow wave discharges with maximal amplitude in frontal lobes and poor organization of background activity. At 10 years, the Peabody Picture Vocabulary Test-IV (PPVT-IV) revealed markedly low verbal abilities (verbal age 4 years and 4 months). An attempt to withdraw valproic acid at 10 years increased epileptic activity. Currently, the patient is 12 years old, and she has adapted to a mainstream school with the support of special education teachers and speech therapy. She suffers from occasional partial and secondarily generalized tonic-clonic seizures. Background activity on EEG recording has normalized, and no paroxysms are registered.

Biochemical and Genetic Studies

As part of a screening for inborn errors of metabolism, purines and pyrimidines were analyzed in urine and plasma. Strongly elevated concentrations of uracil and thymine were observed in urine and plasma which suggested that the patient had a DPD deficiency (Table 1). Subsequent analysis showed no residual DPD activity in peripheral blood mononuclear cells. Sequence analysis of *DPYD* showed that the patient was homozygous for the c.257C > T (p.Pro86Leu) variant (Table 1). Expression of the mutant *DPYD* construct containing the c.257C > T (p.Pro86Leu) variant in HEK293 Flp-In cells showed that the DPD mutant carrying the Pro86Leu variant possessed hardly any residual activity (0.7%) compared to the wild-type enzyme (Fig. 1). To exclude the possibility that the lack of DPD activity was the result of an inability to produce the mutant DPD protein in HEK293 Flp-In cells, the DPD protein expression levels were analyzed by immunoblotting. Figure 1 shows that the mutant DPD protein, carrying the Pro86Leu variant, was expressed in a comparable amount as the wild-type protein. Thus, the lack of DPD activity of the mutant DPD enzyme in HEK293 Flp-In cells is not due to rapid degradation of the mutant DPD protein in the HEK293 Flp-In lysates.

DNA sequence analysis in the father demonstrated that he was heterozygous for the c.257C > T variant in *DPYD*, but in the mother the variant could not be detected. *DPYD* is prone to acquire genomic rearrangements due to the presence of an intragenic fragile site *FRA1E*, but MLPA analysis showed no intragenic deletions or amplifications of *DPYD* in the patient or parents. Haplotype analyses with 26

Table 1 Biochemical and genetic analysis of a DPD-deficient patient

| Subject | Urine (μmol/mmol creatinine) | | Plasma (μM) | | DPD activity [nmol/(mg total protein · h)] | DPYD[a] |
	Uracil	Thymine	Uracil	Thymine		
Patient	236	131	13.4	15.2	<0.025	c.257[C > T];[C > T]
Father	n.a.	n.a.	n.a.	n.a.	n.a.	c.257[C > T];[=]
Mother	n.a.	n.a.	n.a.	n.a.	n.a.	c.257C=
Controls					9.9 ± 2.8 (n = 54)[b]	
Median	5	<1	0.19	0.04		
Range	1–35 (n = 112)	<1 (n = 112)	0.08–0.36 (n = 100)	0.02–0.09 (n = 100)		

n.a. not available

[a] Nomenclature according to http://varnomen.hgvs.org/

[b] Data taken from (van Kuilenburg et al. 2002b)

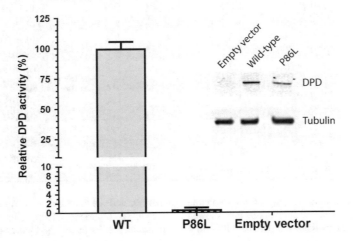

Fig. 1 DPD activity and immunoblot analysis of recombinantly expressed wild-type and mutant DPD enzymes. The results represent the relative DPD activity (mean + SD, n = 3) of the DPD mutant carrying the Pro86Leu variant compared to wild-type DPD enzyme. The insert shows the immunoblot analysis of the expressed wild-type and mutant DPD enzyme

microsatellite repeats distributed over chromosome 1 to probe for homozygosity for the c.257C > T variant in *DPYD* by uniparental isodisomy for chromosome 1 demonstrated the patient to be homozygous for all 26 markers (Fig. 2). Fourteen markers were uninformative since they could have been inherited from either parent. For one marker only paternal uniparental disomy (UPD) could be proven. Paternal isodisomy was observed for 11 markers (Fig. 2).

Discussion

Dihydropyrimidine dehydrogenase (DPD) deficiency is an autosomal recessive disease characterized by thymine-uraciluria in homozygous-deficient patients. Here, we present the first case of DPD deficiency due to uniparental isodisomy. The phenotype in the patient, i.e., cognitive impairment, language delay, and seizures, is similar to the

phenotype typically observed in clinically affected patients with DPD deficiency (van Kuilenburg et al. 1999, 2002a, 2009). The MRI findings in the present patient are nonspecific and have been reported infrequently in DPD-deficient patients (Chen et al. 2014; Enns et al. 2004). Chromosome 1 is not known to contain imprinted areas or imprinted genes, so UPD of chromosome 1 is not expected to cause a phenotype by a disturbed methylation.

The frequency of UPD in newborn is considered to be 1 in 3,500–5,000 (Liehr 2010). Chromosomes 7, 11, 14, 15, and 16 are most often involved in uniparental isodisomy formation, and for chromosome 1 only, a moderate frequency of uniparental isodisomy has been observed (Liehr 2010). The c.257C > T variant (rs568132506) is extremely rare in the general population (allele frequency 5.4×10^{-5} in gnomAD; http://gnomad.broadinstitute.org/variant/1-98206012-G-A). So far, this variant has been described in only one patient with a complete DPD

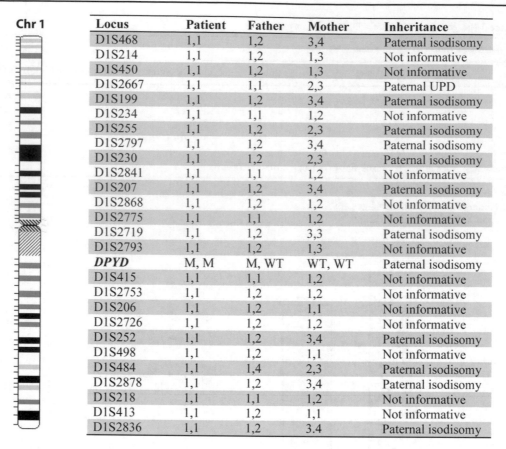

Fig. 2 Genotype analysis of chromosome 1 using 26 microsatellite repeats. The patient was homozygous for all 26 markers and showed paternal uniparental isodisomy for 11 markers and paternal UPD for 1 marker, and 14 markers were uninformative. The presence of the c.257C > T variant (M) or wild-type sequence (WT) of *DPYD* is indicated for the patient and parents

deficiency (van Kuilenburg et al. 2002a). Analysis of the crystal structure of DPD showed that Pro86 is in close proximity to one of the iron-sulfur clusters in the N-terminal domain (van Kuilenburg et al. 2002a). The introduction of a leucine at this position would interfere with the binding of the iron-sulfur cluster, thereby inhibiting electron transport and thus activity (van Kuilenburg et al. 2002a).

The elucidation of genetic mechanisms underlying DPD deficiency is increasingly being appreciated since DPD deficiency has been recognized as an important determinant of fluoropyrimidine-associated toxicity in cancer patients (van Kuilenburg et al. 2017; van Kuilenburg 2004). To date, many pathogenic variants have been described in *DPYD*, and additional rare variants may collectively explain an appreciable fraction of patients with DPD deficiency. Therefore, the identification of novel genetic mechanisms underlying DPD deficiency will not only allow analysis of genotype-phenotype relationships in DPD-deficient patients but also screening of cancer patients at risk. Our study showed that uniparental isodisomy should be considered in DPD-deficient patients with only one parent being a carrier for a pathogenic variant in *DPYD*.

Synopsis

The c.257C > T (p.Pro86Leu) variant in *DPYD* results in a mutant DPD enzyme without residual activity, and uniparental isodisomy should be considered in DPD-deficient patients with only one parent being a carrier for a pathogenic variant in *DPYD*.

Compliance with Ethics Guidelines

Conflict of Interest

André van Kuilenburg, Judith Meijer, Rutger Meinsma, Belén Pérez-Dueñas, Marielle Alders, Zahurul A. Bhuiyan, Rafael Artuch, and Raoul Hennekam declare that they have no conflict of interest.

Details of Ethical Approval

The study (W16_179 # 16.210) was approved by the Medical Ethics Committee of the Academic Medical Center.

Patient Consent Statement

All procedures followed were in accordance with the ethical standards of the responsible committee on human experimentation (institutional) and with the Helsinki Declaration of 1975, as revised in 2000. Informed consent was obtained from the parents of the child included in this study for publication.

Authors' Contribution

André van Kuilenburg and Raoul Hennekam: study design, data analysis, and drafting of the article

Judith Meijer, Rutger Meinsma, Marielle Alders, and Zahurul A. Bhuiyan: experimental data acquisition and data analysis

Belén Pérez-Dueñas and Rafael Artuch: patient care and drafting of the article

Guarantor and Corresponding Author

André B.P. van Kuilenburg accepts full responsibility for the work and conduct of the study, had access to the data, and controlled the decision to publish.

Details of Funding

None

References

Chen BC, Mohd Rawi R, Meinsma R, Meijer J, Hennekam RC, van Kuilenburg AB (2014) Dihydropyrimidine dehydrogenase deficiency in two Malaysian siblings with abnormal MRI findings. Mol Syndromol 5(6):299–303

Enns GM, Barkovich AJ, van Kuilenburg ABP et al (2004) Head imaging abnormalities in dihydropyrimidine dehydrogenase deficiency. J Inherit Metab Dis 27(4):513–522

Fleger M, Willomitzer J, Meinsma R et al (2017) Dihydropyrimidine dehydrogenase deficiency: metabolic disease or biochemical phenotype? JIMD Rep 37:49–54

Johnson MR, Diasio RB (2001) Importance of dihydropyrimidine dehydrogenase (DPD) deficiency in patients exhibiting toxicity following treatment with 5-fluorouracil. Adv Enzyme Regul 41:151–157

Liehr T (2010) Cytogenetic contribution to uniparental disomy (UPD). Mol Cytogenet 3:8

van Kuilenburg ABP (2004) Dihydropyrimidine dehydrogenase and the efficacy and toxicity of 5-fluorouracil. Eur J Cancer 40 (7):939–950

van Kuilenburg ABP, Vreken P, Abeling NGGM et al (1999) Genotype and phenotype in patients with dihydropyrimidine dehydrogenase deficiency. Hum Genet 104(1):1–9

van Kuilenburg ABP, Dobritzsch D, Meinsma JR et al (2002a) Novel disease-causing mutations in the dihydropyrimidine dehydrogenase gene interpreted by analysis of the three-dimensional protein structure. Biochem J 364(Pt 1):157–163

van Kuilenburg ABP, Meinsma JR, Zoetekouw L, van Gennip AH (2002b) Increased risk of grade IV neutropenia after administration of 5-fluorouracil due to a dihydropyrimidine dehydrogenase deficiency: high prevalence of the IVS14+1g>a mutation. Int J Cancer 101(3):253–258

van Kuilenburg ABP, Meijer J, Mul ANP et al (2009) Analysis of severely affected patients with dihydropyrimidine dehydrogenase deficiency reveals large intragenic rearrangements of DPYD and a de novo interstitial deletion del(1)(p13.3p21.3). Hum Genet 125(5–6):581–590

van Kuilenburg AB, Meijer J, Maurer D et al (2017) Severe fluoropyrimidine toxicity due to novel and rare DPYD missense mutations, deletion and genomic amplification affecting DPD activity and mRNA splicing. Biochim Biophys Acta 1863 (3):721–730

van Lenthe H, van Kuilenburg ABP, Ito T et al (2000) Defects in pyrimidine degradation identified by HPLC-electrospray tandem mass spectrometry of urine specimens or urine-soaked filter paper strips. Clin Chem 46(12):1916–1922

Wei X, Elizondo G, Sapone A et al (1998) Characterization of the human dihydropyrimidine dehydrogenase gene. Genomics 51 (3):391–400

JIMD Reports
DOI 10.1007/8904_2018_143

Severe Neonatal Manifestations of Infantile Liver Failure Syndrome Type 1 Caused by Cytosolic Leucine-tRNA Synthetase Deficiency

Christina Peroutka · Jacqueline Salas ·
Jacquelyn Britton · Juliet Bishop · Lisa Kratz ·
Maureen M. Gilmore · Jill A. Fahrner ·
W. Christopher Golden · Tao Wang

Received: 23 July 2018 / Revised: 12 September 2018 / Accepted: 14 September 2018 / Published online: 23 October 2018
© Society for the Study of Inborn Errors of Metabolism (SSIEM) 2018

Abstract *Background*: Deleterious mutations in cytosolic leucine-tRNA synthetase (LARS) cause infantile liver failure syndrome, type 1 (ILFS1), a recently recognized, rare autosomal recessive disorder (OMIM151350). Only six families with ILFS1 have been reported in the literature. Patients with ILFS1 are typically diagnosed between 5 and 24 months of age with failure to thrive, developmental delays, encephalopathy, microcytic anemia, and chronic liver dysfunction with recurrent exacerbations following childhood illnesses. Neonatal manifestations of this disorder have not been well documented.

Case Report: We report a premature female newborn with intrauterine growth restriction, failure to thrive, congenital anemia, anasarca, and fulminant liver failure leading to lethal multiple organ failure. Liver failure in this infant was characterized by a disproportionate impairment of liver synthetic function, including severe coagulopathy and hypoalbuminemia without significant defects in liver detoxification or evidence of hepatocellular injury during early phase of the disease. Whole-exome sequencing of child-parent trio identified two inherited missense mutations in *LARS* in this patient. One, c.1292T>A;

p.Val431Asp, has been reported in patients with ILFS1, while the other, c.725C>T; p.Pro242Leu, is novel. Both mutations involve amino acid residues in the highly conserved editing domain of LARS, are predicted to be functionally deleterious, and presumably contribute to the clinical manifestations in this patient.

Conclusion: This is the first case documenting neonatal manifestation of ILFS1, highlighting early, severe, and disproportionate defects in liver synthetic function. Timely diagnosis of ILFS1 is crucial to guide critical clinical management and improve outcomes of this rare and potentially life-threatening disorder.

Communicated by: John Christodoulou, MB BS PhD FRACP FRCPA

C. Peroutka · J. Salas · M. M. Gilmore · J. A. Fahrner ·
W. C. Golden (✉) · T. Wang (✉)
Department of Pediatrics, Johns Hopkins University School of
Medicine, Baltimore, MD, USA
e-mail: cgolden@jhmi.edu; twang9@jhmi.edu

C. Peroutka · J. Britton · J. Bishop · L. Kratz · J. A. Fahrner · T. Wang
Institute of Genetic Medicine, Johns Hopkins University School of
Medicine, Baltimore, MD, USA

L. Kratz
Kennedy Krieger Institute, Baltimore, MD, USA

Introduction

Neonatal acute liver failure (NALF) is a rare and poorly understood disease entity (Taylor and Whitington 2016; Bitar et al. 2017). Determining the etiology of NALF presents a unique and urgent clinical challenge given extensive differential diagnoses and often rapid and fulminant disease progression (Sundaram et al. 2011). Establishing a timely diagnosis is critical to guiding clinical management, as many NALF disorders are medically and/or surgically treatable with favorable outcomes (Bitar et al. 2017; Sundaram et al. 2011; Devictor et al. 2011).

LARS encodes cytosolic leucine-tRNA synthetase, an enzyme critical for incorporating leucine (the most abundant amino acid) during protein synthesis. Deleterious mutations in *LARS* cause infantile liver failure syndrome, type 1 (ILFS1), a recently recognized, rare autosomal recessive disorder (OMIM151350). Only six families have been reported in the literature, with the majority of affected individuals from the Irish Traveller population (Casey et al. 2012, 2015; El-Gharbawy et al. 2015; Lin et al. 2017). Reported patients have been diagnosed between 5 and 24 months of age, with variable clinical phenotypes, including liver dysfunction with recurrent exacerbations, microcytic anemia, failure to thrive, encephalopathy, developmental delays, and intellectual disability. Neonatal manifestations of this disorder have not been well documented.

We report a case of a premature female neonate who presented with intrauterine growth restriction (IUGR), congenital anemia, anasarca, and fulminant liver failure who was found to be a compound heterozygote for two deleterious mutations in *LARS*. This is the first report documenting severe neonatal manifestations of ILFS1 and highlights defects in liver synthetic function as an initial presentation of this rare and potentially lethal genetic disorder.

Case Report

This female infant was born at 29–6/7 weeks of gestation by Cesarean section in the setting of intrauterine growth restriction and maternal preeclampsia. Maternal history was significant for two prior first-trimester pregnancy losses of unknown etiology and a threatened first-trimester loss in this pregnancy. APGAR scores were 7 and 9 at 1 and 5 min of life, respectively. Physical examination at birth was remarkable for a small for gestational age female (weight 760 g, 5th percentile; length 32 cm, 1st percentile; head circumference 25.5 cm, 18th percentile) with a two-vessel cord. Immediate neonatal course was notable for mild respiratory distress, congenital anemia (hemoglobin 9.1 g/dL; MCV 101.1 fL), transient hyponatremia, and apnea of prematurity. Breast milk feedings were initiated but stopped several times due to abdominal distention. At 25 days of age, the infant developed increased work of breathing, abdominal distention, diffuse edema, hematemesis, and hematochezia. Her laboratory studies showed coagulopathy and hypoalbuminemia; her abdominal imaging demonstrated bowel wall thickening and moderate ascites. She was stabilized on mechanical ventilation and treated with empiric antibiotics.

Head ultrasound showed mild asymmetric prominence of the left lateral ventricle without hemorrhage. Abdominal ultrasound showed increasing echogenicity of the right kidney, intermittent reversal of blood flow within the main portal vein, reversal of blood flow within the left portal vein, and moderate ascites, but without significant hepatosplenomegaly. Echocardiography showed pulmonary hypertension, a small muscular ventricular septum defect, and normal biventricular function. Exploratory laparotomy (performed due to a concern for necrotizing enterocolitis) demonstrated approximately 30 mL of clear ascites but no evidence of bowel necrosis or malrotation. A catheterized urine specimen showed moderate leukocyte esterase and grew *Candida lusitaniae* at 3 days; the patient was treated with 14 days of intravenous fluconazole. Evaluations for causes of infectious hepatitis, including herpes simplex virus, cytomegalovirus, enterovirus, parvovirus, and hepatitis B and C, were negative.

During her hospital course, laboratory studies showed persistent anemia (nadir 7.9 g/dL; normal 14.1–20.1 g/dL) despite several packed red cell transfusions and hypoalbuminemia (1.5–2.8 g/dL; normal, 3.5–5.3 g/dL) refractory to multiple albumin transfusions and protein intake of up to 3.5 g/kg/day from total parenteral nutrition. She had severe coagulopathy (PT 16.5–44.9 s [normal 10.0–13.6 s]; PTT 34.2–166.4 s [normal 26.9–62.5 s]; INR 1.6–4.6 [normal 0.86–1.22]). Plasma ammonia levels were normal (55–129 μmol/L; normal <150 μmol/L). Serum bilirubin levels were mildly elevated (peak total bilirubin 6.3 mg/dL; peak direct bilirubin 4.6 mg/dL) at 29 days of life, and serum transaminases were normal to borderline elevated: aspartate aminotransferase (26–99 IU/L; normal <31 IU/L), alanine aminotransferase (7–68 IU/L; normal <31 IU/L), and γ-glutamyltransferase (23–27 U/L; normal 12–123 U/L). As her illness progressed, she developed thrombocytopenia (nadir 23 K/mL; normal 180–327 K/mL), low factor VII activity (5%; normal >25%), low fibrinogen level (47 mg/dL; normal 82–383 mg/dL), and elevated D-dimer (6.42–7.55 mg/L FEU; normal 0.11–0.42 mg/L FEU), which did not correct after multiple fresh frozen plasma and cryoprecipitate transfusions. Despite maximal ventilation support, aggressive treatment of infection, and optimized nutrition, she developed severe respiratory failure, vasopressor-refractory hypotension, renal failure, and profound anasarca. She died due to multi-organ failure at 53 days of age.

The infant had an elevated immunoreactive trypsinogen (IRT level >468 ng/mL; normal <100 ng/mL) on her initial state newborn screen. However, molecular testing for 23 common mutations for cystic fibrosis (core pathogenic mutations recommended by American College of Medical Genetics) was negative, and a repeat IRT also was normal. Her serum lactate levels were intermittently elevated (4–6.9 mmol/L; normal, 0.5–2.2 mmol/L). Total and fractionated carnitine levels and acylcarnitine profile did not suggest a known inborn error of metabolism. Plasma amino acids showed nonspecific moderate elevation of several amino acids including tyrosine (361–748 μmol/L; normal 20–108 μmol/L), methionine (96–148 μmol/L; normal 7–43 μmol/L), and glycine (745–927 μmol/L; normal 87–323 μmol/L). Urine organic acids showed increased excretion of 4-hydroxyphenyllactate and 4-hydroxyphenylpyruvate, suggesting either liver immaturity or dysfunction. Quantitative blood succinylacetone was normal (1.9 nmol/mL; normal <5 nmol/mL). Carbohydrate-deficient transferrin electrophoresis showed a normal profile. Alpha-fetoprotein levels were age-appropriate (6,964–11,601 ng/mL; normal <22,062 ng/mL). Serum ferritin levels were normal to borderline elevated (314–952 ng/mL; normal 200–600 ng/mL).

A single nucleotide polymorphism (SNP) microarray identified an 807 kb interstitial duplication at 17p12 of unknown clinical significance which was inherited from her mother who is asymptomatic. Mitochondrial DNA sequencing and deletion/duplication analysis found no pathogenic variants. Whole-exome sequencing utilizing the child-parent trio revealed compound heterozygosity in the infant for two potentially pathogenic variants in *LARS* [NM_020117.9] (Fig. 1). One missense variant, c.1292T>A; p.Val431Asp in exon 14 [NM_020117.9], was maternally inherited, has a cumulative allele frequency of 0.0003612, and has not been observed in a homozygous state in large population cohorts (gnomad.broadinstitute.org). This amino acid substitution is located in the LARS editing domain crucial to protein function (Fig. 1) (Han et al. 2012; Huang et al. 2014) and occurs at a position where only amino acids with similar properties to valine (isoleucine and leucine) appear tolerated across species. In silico analysis indicates that amino acid substitution of valine by aspartate results in significant changes in polarity, charge, and size of the residue and predicts a probably damaging effect on protein structure and/or function [PolyPhen-2: 0.994; probably damaging (http://genetics.bwh.harvard.edu/pph2/) and CADD-PHRED: 29.5 https://cadd.gs.washington.edu/)]. Importantly, this variant has been previously described in two unrelated, non-Irish Traveller patients with ILFS1 (El-Gharbawy et al. 2015). Five of the eight previously reported mutations in ILFS1 patients are located in this LARS editing domain (Fig. 1). The second missense variant, c.725C>T; p.Pro242Leu in

exon 8 [NM_020117.9], was paternally inherited, has a cumulative allele frequency of 0.00001628, and has not been observed in a homozygous state in large population cohorts (gnomad.broadinstitute.org). This amino acid substitution is located in the CH1 hairpin motif of the editing domain of LARS at an amino acid position that is highly conserved across species (Fig. 1) (Lin et al. 2017). In silico analysis predicts that it is probably damaging to protein structure and/or function (PolyPhen-2: 0.998; probably damaging; CADD-PHRED: 32). This novel variant has not been reported previously in ILFS1. Subsequent testing confirmed that a healthy 3-year-old sister of this patient is heterozygous for this variant.

Discussion

ILFS1 is a newly recognized, rare autosomal recessive disorder caused by deleterious mutations in *LARS*. Patients typically present from infancy to early childhood during periods of illness or other physiological stress. Noted clinical features include preterm delivery, intrauterine growth restriction, failure to thrive, microcytic anemia, hypoalbuminemia, coagulopathy, recurrent liver dysfunction, liver fibrosis and cirrhosis, renal dysfunction, encephalopathy, developmental delays, and intellectual disability (Table 1). Chronic liver dysfunction with intermittent exacerbations (triggered by fever, infection, and physical and/or metabolic stress conditions) leads to progressive liver failure, fibrosis, and cirrhosis (Table 1). In addition to premature birth, IUGR, and congenital anemia, our patient presented with a fulminant course of liver failure leading to multi-organ failure. This case provides valuable clues for initial recognition and underscores importance of early diagnosis of this potentially lethal genetic disorder. Although available genetic findings and core clinical manifestations of this patient are consistent with ILFS1,

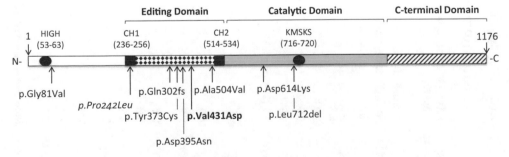

Fig. 1 Cytosolic leucine-tRNA synthetase domains and mutations found in ILFS1 patients. Brackets indicate the editing, catalytic, and c-terminal domains of human cytosolic leucine-tRNA synthetase. The HIGH motif is the ATP binding site; CH1 and CH2 represent CP1 hairpin 1 and 2; KMSKS is the mobile pentapeptide motif regulating conformational changes of tRNA synthetase, with amino acid position

of each motif in parentheses. *c.725C>T; p.Pro242Leu* (novel) is the paternal variant for this patient and is *italicized*. **c.1292T>A; p.Val431Asp** (previously reported) is the maternal variant for this patient marked in **bold**. All other variants are previously reported variants

Table 1 Clinical features of reported patients with infantile liver failure syndrome type 1 caused by cytosolic leucine-tRNA synthetase deficiency

Source	Casey et al. (2012, 2015)	Casey et al. (2015)	El-Gharbawy et al. (2015)	El-Gharbawy et al. (2015)	Lin et al. (2017)	Current report
Ethnicity	Irish Travellers	Ashkenazi Jewish	Caucasian, non-Irish Traveller	Caucasian, non-Irish Traveller	Chinese	Caucasian, non-Irish Traveller
No. of reported families (no. of patients)	2 (9)	1 (1)	1 (1)	1 (1)	1 (1)	1 (1)
Variant 1	c.1118A>G; p.Tyr373Cys	c.1511C>T; p.Ala504Val	c. 242G>T; p.Gly81Val	c.903delG; p.Gln302fs	c.1183G>A; p.Asp395Asn	c.725C>T; p.Pro242Leu
Variant 2	c.1118A>G; p.Tyr373Cys	c.1842C>G; p.Asp614Lys	c.1292T>A; p.Val431Asp	c.1292T>A; p.Val431Asp	c.2133_2135del; p.Leu712del	c.1292T>A; p.Val431Asp
In silico analysis with PolyPhen-2; prediction (score)	p.Tyr373Cys; damaging (0.993)	NR	NR	NR	p.Asp395Asn; damaging (0.999)	p.Pro242Leu; probably damaging (0.998) p.Val431Asp; probably damaging (0.994)
Age at presentation	1 month–2 years	5 months	17 months	13 months	18 months	Neonatal (<1 month)
Sex (no. individuals)	Male (7); female (2)	Female	Female	Male	Male	Female
Pregnancy complications	NR	NR	Recurrent pregnancy loss	Recurrent pregnancy loss; HELLP	NR	Recurrent pregnancy loss; preeclampsia
Premature birth	6/9	NR	Y	Y	N	Y
Low birth weight	9/9	Y	NR	NR	Y	Y
Failure to thrive	9/9	Y	Y	NR	Y	Y
Microcytic anemia	7/9	Y	Y	NR	Y	Y
Acute liver failure (age of first episode)	5/9 (2–8 months)	Y (5 months)	Y (17 months)	NR	NR	Y (<1 month)
Intermittent liver dysfunction (within first year)	4/9	NR	NR	Y	Y	Y
Hypoalbuminemia	9/9	Y	NR	NR	Y	Y
Coagulopathy (elevated PT/PTT/INR)	9/9	Y	Y	Y	Y	Y
Hyperbilirubinemia	9/9	Y	NR	Y	Y	Y
Hepatomegaly	3/9	NR	NR	NR	Y	N
Hepatic steatosis	4/4	NR	Y	Hepatic necrosis	Y	NR
Liver fibrosis, nodules, cirrhosis	2/4	NR	Y	NR	Y	NR
Developmental delays	8/9	Y	NR	Y	NR	NR
Seizure disorders	9/9	Y	NR	NR	NR	N
Renal failure or Fanconi syndrome	2/9	NR	Y	NR	NR	Y
Brain imaging studies	Mild cerebral atrophy 4/7	Stroke	NR	NR	NR	Asymmetric prominence of the left lateral ventricle
Other biochemical genetic testing[a]	Negative	Negative	Negative	Elevation of plasma tyrosine	Negative	Elevation of plasma tyrosine
Additional notes						Ascites; anasarca; DIC

Y yes/present, N no/absent, NR not reported, DIC disseminated intravascular coagulation, HELLP hemolysis, elevated liver enzymes, and low platelets, INR international normalized ratio, PT prothrombin time, PTT partial thromboplastin time

[a] Targeted biochemical testing such as plasma amino acids, urine organic acids, succinylacetone, acylcarnitine profile, and fractionated carnitine

functional characterizations of these variants are warranted to establish a definitive causal relationship.

Prematurity, IUGR, and anemia are relatively nonspecific findings commonly seen in neonates admitted to the neonatal intensive care unit (NICU). Impaired liver function (with elevated transaminases and γ-glutamyl transferase, hyperbilirubinemia, hyperammonemia, hypoglycemia, hypoalbuminemia, and coagulopathy in neonates) can be caused by infectious hepatitis, gestational alloimmune liver disease, histophagocytic lymphohistocytosis, systematic illnesses (such as hypoxia and sepsis), and metabolic disorders (including tyrosinemia type I, galactosemia, alpha-1-antitrypsin deficiency, and mitochondrial disorders). In the majority of these disorders, hepatocellular injury results in elevated transaminases and, ultimately, defects in liver detoxification and liver synthetic function. Although ILFS1 patients develop recurrent hepatic dysfunction leading to progressive liver fibrosis and cirrhosis with disease progression, this case highlights the disproportionately impaired liver synthetic function causing severe and persistent coagulopathy and hypoalbuminemia during early course of the disease. In our patient, liver transaminases and γ-glutamyltransferase were normal or only mildly elevated, suggesting absence of significant hepatocyte and biliary tree injury. Additionally, liver detoxification functions of ammonia, bilirubin, and bile acids were normal or only mildly affected. This liver failure profile, coupled with congenital anemia, prenatal and postnatal growth restriction, and negative evaluations for other common causes of neonatal liver failure, serves as a valuable clue for early diagnosis of ILFS1 during the neonatal period. Additionally, early WES-based diagnosis could potentially establish or eliminate inborn errors of metabolism and other genetic disorders presenting with neonatal liver failure and reduce expansive diagnostic workups. Data from WES analysis also may provide neonatologists and pediatric critical care specialists with prognostic and therapeutic guidance in managing such diseases. In ILFS-1, for example, initiation of early, aggressive nutrition support has been proposed to benefit affected patients (El-Gharbawy et al. 2015).

The pathophysiology of LARS deficiency is incompletely understood. The failure to incorporate leucine efficiently during protein synthesis is particularly detrimental to organs that depend on high-protein synthesis rate (such as the liver and bone marrow) during periods of rapid physical growth in infancy and early childhood. We speculate that this mechanism contributes to the observed intrauterine growth restriction and failure to thrive in ILFS1 patients. This mechanism also may in part explain why clinical symptoms are improved in ILFS1 patients during later adolescence and adulthood when physical growth and demands for protein synthesis slow down. Consistent with this mechanism, tissues with high demand for protein synthesis, such as liver, hematopoietic cells, and immune systems, are commonly affected in ILFS1 patients (Casey et al. 2012, 2015; El-Gharbawy et al. 2015; Lin et al. 2017). Finally, recent studies showed that LARS functions as a leucine sensor in regulating the mTORC1-signaling pathway, which plays a key role in many cellular processes, including autophagy, and cell growth (Han et al. 2012).

Only six families with ILFS1 were reported in the literature (Table 1). Two families, including the original family with eight patients, are Irish Travellers (Casey et al. 2012, 2015). However, current literature supports an expanding awareness of ILFS1 in populations outside of this group. *LARS* mutations have been found in unrelated ILFS1 patients of Ashkenazi Jewish, Caucasian non-Irish Traveller, and Chinese descent (Casey et al. 2015; El-Gharbawy et al. 2015; Lin et al. 2017) (Table 1). LARS deficiency-related ILFS1 likely is under-recognized for several reasons. Early clinical features such as IUGR, failure to thrive, anemia, and liver dysfunction are relatively nonspecific in premature infants. In older children, ILFS1 exacerbations are often triggered by common childhood illnesses such as fever and systematic infection, and the associated hepatic and red cell abnormalities may be attributed to the illness itself. Thus, high clinical vigilance is needed to recognize the profile of ILFS1 manifestations at different ages leading to early diagnosis and optimized treatment to achieve desirable clinical outcomes and prevent permanent liver damage and other severe complications.

Though specific treatment to ILFS1 is not yet available, patients with ILFS1 should be admitted, even with minor illnesses, for aggressive treatment and supportive care of the underlying causes of physical and/or metabolic stress. High dextrose infusions (to suppress catabolism) and sufficient protein intake (to promote protein synthesis) are indicated during acute exacerbations to minimize liver damage and reduce risks of complications involving multi-organs (Casey et al. 2015; El-Gharbawy et al. 2015).

Details of the Contributions of Individual Authors

Christina M. Peroutka, Jacqueline L. Salas, Juliet Bishop, and Jacquelyn F. Britton contributed to collection, analyses, and interpretation of data and drafting the article. W. Christopher Golden, Maureen M. Gilmore, Lisa Kratz, Jill A. Fahrner, and Tao Wang contributed to conception and design, data analysis and interpretation, and drafting the article or revising it critically for important intellectual content.

All authors read and approved the final manuscript.

Details of Funding

C.M.P. and J.C.B. are supported by NIH grant T32GM007471 awarded to the Johns Hopkins University.

Ethics Statement

This study is in accordance with the ethical standards of the responsible conduct on human subject research (institutional and national) and with the Helsinki Declaration of 1975, as revised in 2000.

Parental Consent

The authors obtained parental consent to use protected health information presented in this report.

Synopsis

The triad of congenital anemia, prenatal and postnatal growth restriction, and severely impaired liver synthetic functions are early neonatal manifestation of infantile liver failure syndrome 1 caused by a deficiency of cytosolic leucine-tRNA synthetase.

Compliance with Ethics Guidelines

Christina Peroutka, Jacqueline Salas, Jacquelyn Britton, Juliet Bishop, Lisa Kratz, Maureen M. Gilmore, Jill Fahrner, W. Christopher Golden, and Tao Wang declare that they have no conflict of interest.

References

Bitar R, Thwaites R, Davison S et al (2017) Liver failure in early infancy: aetiology, presentation, and outcome. J Pediatr Gastroenterol Nutr 64:70–75

Casey J, McGettigan P, Lynam-Lennon N et al (2012) Identification of a mutation in LARS as a novel cause of infantile hepatopathy. Mol Genet Metab 106:351–358

Casey J, Slattery S, Cotter M et al (2015) Clinical and genetic characterisation of infantile liver failure syndrome type 1, due to recessive mutations in LARS. J Inherit Metab Dis 38:1085–1092

Devictor D, Tissieres P, Durand P et al (2011) Acute liver failure in neonates, infants and children. Expert Rev Gastroenterol Hepatol 5:717–729

El-Gharbawy A, Sebastian J, Ghaloul-Gonzalez L, Mroczkowski J, Goldstein A, Venkat V, Dobrowolski S, Squires R, Vockley J (2015) LARS mutations in non-Irish travelers: an under-recognized multi-system disorder characterized by infantile hepatopathy during physiological stress. Mitochondrion 24 (Suppl):S40–S41

Han J, Jeong S, Park M et al (2012) Leucyl-tRNA synthetase is an intracellular leucine sensor for the mTORC1-signaling pathway. Cell 149:410–424

Huang Q, Zhou X, Hu Q et al (2014) A bridge between the aminoacylation and editing domains of leucyl-tRNA synthetase is crucial for its synthetic activity. RNA 20:1440–1450

Lin W, Zheng Q, Guo L, Cheng Y, Song YZ (2017) First non-Caucasian case of infantile liver failure syndrome type I: clinical characteristics and molecular diagnosis. Chin J Contemp Pediatr 19:913–920. https://doi.org/10.7499/j.issn.1008-8830.2017.08.013

Sundaram S, Alonso E, Narkewicz M et al (2011) Characterization and outcomes of young infants with acute liver failure. J Pediatr 159:813–818

Taylor S, Whitington P (2016) Neonatal acute liver failure. Liver Transpl 22:677–685

JIMD Reports
DOI 10.1007/8904_2018_141

RESEARCH REPORT

Enzyme Replacement Therapy in Pregnant Women with Fabry Disease: A Case Series

Pehuén Fernández · Shunko Oscar Fernández ·
Jacqueline Griselda Mariela Gonzalez ·
Tabaré Fernández · Cinthia Claudia Fernández ·
Segundo Pastor Fernández

Received: 11 May 2018 / Revised: 27 August 2018 / Accepted: 30 August 2018 / Published online: 08 November 2018
© Society for the Study of Inborn Errors of Metabolism (SSIEM) 2018

Abstract Fabry disease is a rare inherited lysosomal
storage disorder caused by the deficiency of the enzyme
alpha-galactosidase A. There is uncertainty regarding the
safety of enzyme replacement therapy during pregnancy.
We describe the course and outcome of seven pregnancies
in six patients with Fabry disease who continued or
reinitiated enzyme replacement therapy during pregnancy.
No adverse events, in both mothers and children, were
observed.

Introduction

Fabry disease (FD) is a rare X-linked lysosomal storage
disorder caused by the deficiency of the enzyme alpha-
galactosidase A (α-Gal A). This condition results in the
accumulation of glycosphingolipids, mainly globotriaosylceramide (gb3), in the lysosomes of cells throughout the
body (Germain 2010) and impairs the function of major
organs, including the heart, the kidneys, and the central and
peripheral nervous systems, often leading to death at an
early age (Tuttolomondo et al. 2013).

Communicated by: Carla E. Hollak, M.D.

We describe the course and outcome of seven pregnancies in six
patients with Fabry disease who received enzyme replacement therapy
during their pregnancies and lactation, without reporting any adverse
events.

P. Fernández (✉) · S. O. Fernández · J. G. M. Gonzalez ·
T. Fernández · C. C. Fernández · S. P. Fernández
CIDTEF, Centro de Investigación, Diagnóstico y Tratamiento de
Enfermedad de Fabry (Research, Diagnosis and Treatment Center for
Fabry Disease), San Fernando del Valle de Catamarca, Argentina
e-mail: pehuenfernandez@hotmail.com

Men with classical FD typically present more severe
clinical manifestations than women and nonclassically
affected male patients. Because of X-chromosome inactivation, women with FD may experience a variable range of
symptoms (Echevarria et al. 2016). The efficacy of enzyme
replacement therapy (ERT) has been demonstrated (Baehner
et al. 2003) among these female patients.

There are few publications addressing the use of ERT in
pregnant women, with only nine cases reported worldwide
treated with agalsidase alfa (Wendt et al. 2005; Dehout
et al. 2006; Kalkum et al. 2009; Hughes et al. 2012). The
largest case series to date was presented by Hughes in
2012, who reported on the administration of ERT during
five pregnancies (Hughes et al. 2012). No experimental
studies specifically assessing drug safety during pregnancy
have been conducted in humans.

Methods

In this series, we retrospectively reviewed the medical
records of all FD patients receiving ERT during pregnancy
and lactation at the *Centro de Investigación, Diagnóstico y
Tratamiento de Enfermedad de Fabry* (CIDTEF, Research,
Diagnosis and Treatment Center for Fabry Disease) in
Catamarca, Argentina, between January 2012 and December 2017. Relevant clinical, laboratory, and imaging
findings are provided for all patients. Data were collected
from each pregnant woman at diagnosis and during the
course of pregnancy and lactation. Baseline characteristics,
including age (in years), mutation of the GLA gene, signs
and symptoms at presentation, activity of the α-Gal A
enzyme, imaging studies, indication, and dose of ERT, were
registered. During pregnancy, age (in years), initiation or
resumption of ERT, potential treatment-emergent adverse
effects and/or complications, mode of administration, and

gestational age at the time of delivery (in weeks) were recorded. For newborns, gender, weight (in grams), length (in centimeters), and Apgar score at birth were recorded, including data on whether or not they were breastfed (exclusively or partially) and for how long (in months), their current age (in years), and subsequent health issues, if any.

To calculate the newborns' weight and height percentiles, international standards were used according to gestational age and sex (Villar et al. 2014).

Results

Six women with FD who received ERT during their pregnancies were included. Patient 3 had two previous pregnancies.

The patients' baseline characteristics are shown in Table 1. All FD diagnoses were made by family screening of the index case. All six patients share the same genetic mutation (exon 3 of the GLA gene coding region c.520T>G, missense-type mutation, C174G genotype, late-onset phenotype). The median age at diagnosis was 22 years old (range 16–35 years). During follow-up, all women showed signs or symptoms of FD. Patient 1 presented mainly with peripheral nervous system involvement (compromise of A-delta fibers in lower limbs) with severe neuropathic pain (acroparesthesias) and heat intolerance that affected her quality of life. The remaining six patients presented kidney involvement, with a decrease in glomerular filtration rate (patients 2, 4, 5, 6) and microalbuminuria (patient 3), confirmed by typical histological

findings of FD in renal biopsies (patients 3, 4, 6). Pain crises occurred in patients 1, 2, and 3. Most patients (1, 2, 4, 5) had reduced activity of the α-Gal A enzyme. All six women had started ERT prior to their pregnancies and received intravenous infusions of agalsidase alfa at a dose of 0.2 mg/kg every 14 days.

The patients' characteristics during pregnancy and the follow-up of their child are shown in Table 2. The median age at the time of pregnancy diagnosis was 26 years old (range 19–38 years). In patients 1, 2, and 3, ERT was discontinued during the first trimester. Given the recurrence of severe untreatable pain crises (pain visual analog scale 8–9/10), it was decided to resume therapy, thereby leading to a major improvement of symptoms. Pregnancy in patient number 4 was confirmed late (Week 10), so ERT was continued. Patients 5 and 6 had impaired renal function and experienced kidney disease progression. The decision to continue ERT was agreed with each patient and their relatives upon the assessment of the risk-benefit balance. All patients underwent close medical follow-up during pregnancy. No drug-related adverse effects were reported.

End of pregnancy occurred between Weeks 36 and 39 of gestational age by means of five vaginal deliveries and two cesarean sections (C-section). Patient number 3 had developed eclampsia at Week 36 during her first pregnancy. She had proteinuria, a hypertensive crisis, and seizures, which led to an emergency C-section, without further complications.

The median newborns' birthweight was 2,890 g (range: 2,370–3,800 g), and the median birth length was 50 cm (range: 46–51 cm). No infant had their weight or size

Table 1 Baseline characteristics of women with Fabry disease at the time of diagnosis

ID	Age (years)	Mutation	Clinical involvement. Enzymatic dosage	Drug dose
1	35	C174G	• Symptoms: acroparesthesia, pain crisis, heat intolerance • Peripheral nervous system: compromise of A-delta fibers in lower limbs • Hearing: moderate mixed hearing loss • Dosage of alpha-galactosidase A: 0.94 μmol/L/h (reference value: 2.10–10.50 μmol/L/h)	Agalsidase alfa 0.2 mg/kg/ 14 days
2	35	C174G	• Symptoms: acroparesthesia, heat intolerance, pain crisis • Renal: creatinine clearance, 71 mL/min × 1.73 m^2 • Dosage of alpha-galactosidase A: 1.27 μmol/L/h (reference value: 2.10–10.50 μmol/l/h)	Agalsidase alfa 0.2 mg/kg/ 14 days
3	22	C174G	• Symptoms: severe pain crisis • Renal: microalbuminuria 240 mg. Biopsy: microvacuoles in visceral and mesangial cells. Ultrasound: parapelvic renal cyst	Agalsidase alfa 0.2 mg/kg/ 14 days
4	16	C174G	• Renal: creatinine clearance: 72 mL/min × 1.73 m^2. Biopsy: glomeruli with intracytoplasmic microvacuoles in some cells. Electron microscopy: podocytes with intracytoplasmic inclusions resembling zebra bodies and myelin figures	Agalsidase alfa 0.2 mg/kg/14 days
5	28	C174G	• Renal: creatinine clearance, 69 mL/min × 1.73 m^2 • Dosage of alpha-galactosidase A: 1.55 μmol/L/h (reference value: 2.10–10.50 μmol/L/h)	Agalsidase alfa 0.2 mg/kg/14 days
6	18	C174G	• Renal: creatinine clearance, 63 mL/min × 1.73 m^2. Biopsy: microvacuolated podocytes with foamy cytoplasm • Dosage of alpha-galactosidase A: 1.17 μmol/L/h (reference value: 2.10–10.50 μmol/L/h)	Agalsidase alfa 0.2 mg/kg/14 days

Table 2 Patients with FD treated with ERT during pregnancy (mother and child)

ID	Age (years)	Drug	AE	PC	Delivery mode	Gestational age (weeks)	Gender	BW, g (perc[a])	BL, cm (perc[a])	Apgar score	BF (months)	Current age (years)	Follow-up
							Child						
1	36	Agalsidase alfa	No	No	VD	37	F	3,800 (97)	46 (10–50)	9/10	P (5)	5	RUTI up to 2 yo No AM
2	38	Agalsidase alfa	No	No	VD	39	M	3,190 (10–50)	50 (50)	8/10	E (12)	3	Normal
3a	24	Agalsidase alfa	No	Eclampsia	CS	36	F	2,370 (10–50)	47 (50)	6/10	No	2	FD
3b	26	Agalsidase alfa	No	No	CS	37	M	2,890 (50)	51 (97)	8/10	E (12)	1	Normal
4	19	Agalsidase alfa	No	No	VD	39	M	3,085 (10–50)	51 (90)	8–9/10	E (12)	1	Normal
5	29	Agalsidase alfa	No	No	VD	39	F	2,730 (10–50)	51 (90)	8–9/10	P (12)	1	Normal
6	22	Agalsidase alfa	No	No	VD	38	F	2,530 (10)	49 (50–90)	8–9/10	P (10)	4	Asthma

AE adverse events, PC pregnancy complications, VD vaginal delivery, CS cesarean section, F female, M male, BW birth weight, BL birth length, perc percentile, BF breastfeeding, E exclusive, P partial, RUTI recurrent urinary tract infection, yo years old, AM anatomical malformations

[a] Percentiles of BW and BL according to Villar J. et al. International standards for newborn weight, length, and head circumference by gestational age and sex: the Newborn Cross-Sectional Study of the INTERGROWTH-21st Project[10]

below the tenth percentile for their gestational age. The first child of patient number 3 (eclampsia and emergency C-section) had a first-minute Apgar score of less than 8 but recovered spontaneously without any resuscitation maneuvers. This was the only non-breastfed child. Three babies were exclusively breastfed for 6 months and continued breastfeeding during the first year. Babies 1, 5, and 6 were partially breastfed for 5, 12, and 10 months, respectively. One girl experienced five episodes of recurrent uncomplicated urinary tract infections in her first 2 years of age. Urine reflux and anatomical malformations were ruled out by renal and urinary tract ultrasound and a cystourethrography. She has not had any recurrent infections to date. Another child had controlled asthma and received treatment with the leukotriene receptor blocker montelukast and inhaled corticosteroids (fluticasone). FD was diagnosed only in newborn 3a by family screening and was ruled out in the remaining six babies by enzyme activity dosage in males and molecular methods in females. Currently, children's median age is 2 years old (range: 1–5 years old), and no health issues potentially associated with the use of ERT during pregnancy and breastfeeding have been reported.

Discussion

In this report, we describe six related patients with FD treated with agalsidase alfa during pregnancy and lactation. They share the same genetic mutation and have different clinical manifestations of FD. Although this mutation is phenotypically characterized by late disease onset, these patients presented early manifestations and therefore received ERT. Two patients (2 and 5) with decreased glomerular filtration rate refused to undergo kidney biopsy. Kidney damage was attributed to FD due to histologically confirmed early renal involvement in their female relatives harboring the same mutation (patients 3, 4, and 6). In patients 2 and 5, there were no clinical signs or symptoms suggestive of other kidney function-impairing conditions.

In all six cases, the decision of whether or not to continue with ERT during pregnancy was challenging. Beck et al. suggested that the medication could be safely used during pregnancy in light of missing evidence on any harmful effect for the mother or the newborn (Beck 2009). Of note, however, this statement was based on only two cases reported worldwide. In our experience, patients presented either disabling clinical symptoms related to the disease that interfered with daily activities or impairment and progression of their kidney disease. The risks and benefits were carefully weighed, and, in agreement with the patients and their families, a decision was made to continue or resume treatment. The medication was well tolerated in all cases, and no ERT-related complications were reported neither in mothers nor in newborns. Although one pregnant woman developed eclampsia, she was at increased risk, with factors including nulliparity, chronic hypertension, and a family history of preeclampsia (Bartsch et al. 2016).

In conclusion, there is limited evidence in current literature on pregnant women with FD treated with agalsidase alfa. At the time of this writing, the total number of women with FD treated during their pregnancies worldwide was 9 (Wendt et al. 2005; Dehout et al. 2006; Kalkum et al. 2009; Hughes et al. 2012), with the largest series (5 patients) belonging to the Fabry Outcomes Survey (FOS) (Hughes et al. 2012). The outcomes of these pregnancies during ERT are promising.

We present the largest series available in the literature to date, raising the total number of pregnant women receiving treatment for FD with agalsidase alfa to 16. In our case series, agalsidase alfa was safe and well tolerated during pregnancy and lactation, with no adverse events reported in mothers and children. Nevertheless, we believe there is still poor evidence to support its universal use among all pregnant women with symptomatic FD.

Conflicts of Interest

The authors received no funding for this work/manuscript.

Compliance with Ethics Guidelines

- Details of the contributions of individual authors:

  - Pehuén Fernández and Shunko Oscar Fernández: planning (conception and design), conduct (analysis and interpretation of data), and reporting (draft and thorough review)
  - Tabaré Fernández, Jacqueline Griselda Mariela Gonzalez, Cinthia Claudia Fernández, and Segundo Pastor Fernández: planning (conception and design), conduct (analysis and interpretation of data), and reporting (thorough review)

- The name of the corresponding author and guarantor: Pehuén Fernández
- Conflict of interest:

  - Tabaré Fernández and Jacqueline Griselda Mariela Gonzalez declare no conflict of interest.
  - Pehuén Fernández and Cinthia Claudia Fernández have received travel reimbursement for symposia attendance from Shire.
  - Shunko Oscar Fernández and Segundo Pastor Fernández have received travel reimbursement for symposia attendance and speaker honoraria from Shire.

- This study did not receive funding.
- Informed consent

- All procedures followed were in accordance with the ethical standards of the responsible committee on human experimentation (institutional and national) and with the Helsinki Declaration of 1975, as revised in 2000. Informed consent was obtained from all patients for being included in the study authorizing the use of their data for this publication.

• This project was approved by the Bioethics Committee of the Hospital Interzonal San Juan Bautista in Catamarca, Argentina.

References

Baehner F, Kampmann C, Whybra C, Miebach E, Wiethoff CM, Beck M (2003) Enzyme replacement therapy in heterozygous females with Fabry disease: results of a phase IIIB study. J Inherit Metab Dis 26(7):617–627

Bartsch E, Medcalf KE, Park AL, Ray JG (2016) Clinical risk factors for pre-eclampsia determined in early pregnancy: systematic review and meta-analysis of large cohort studies. BMJ 353:i1753

Beck M (2009) Agalsidasealfa for the treatment of Fabry disease: new data on clinical efficacy and safety. Expert Opin Biol Ther 9 (2):255–261

Dehout F, Roland D, Henry F, Langlois A, Van Maldergem L (2006) Successful pregnancy in a patient with Fabry disease receiving enzyme replacement therapy. Acta Paediatr 451(95):137–138

Echevarria L, Benistan K, Toussaint A et al (2016) X-chromosome inactivation in female patients with Fabry disease. Clin Genet 89 (1):44–54

Germain DP (2010) Fabry disease. Orphanet J Rare Dis 5(1):30

Hughes D, Deegan P, Romero B, Hollak C, Giugliani R (2012) Pregnancy events in females with Fabry disease in the Fabry Outcome Survey. Mol Genet Metab 105(2):S37

Kalkum G, Macchiella D, Reinke J, Kölbl H, Beck M (2009) Enzyme replacement therapy with agalsidase alfa in pregnant women with Fabry disease. Eur J Obstet Gynecol Reprod Biol 144(1):92–93

Tuttolomondo A, Pecoraro R, Simonetta I, Miceli S, Pinto A, Licata G (2013) Anderson-Fabry disease: a multiorgan disease. Curr Pharm Des 19(33):5974–5996

Villar J, Ismail LC, Victora CG et al (2014) International standards for newborn, weight, and circumference by gestational age and sex: the Newborn Cross-Sectional Study of the INTERGROWTH-21st Project. Lancet 384(9946):857–868

Wendt S, Whybra C, Kampmann C, Teichmann E, Beck M (2005) Successful pregnancy outcome in a patient with Fabrydisease receiving enzyme replacement therapy with agalsidase alfa. J Inherit Metab Dis 28(5):787–788

JIMD Reports
DOI 10.1007/8904_2018_145

RESEARCH REPORT

Survival of a Male Infant with a Familial Xp11.4 Deletion Causing Ornithine Transcarbamylase Deficiency

Molly McPheron · Melissa Lah

Received: 12 February 2018 / Revised: 14 September 2018 / Accepted: 17 September 2018 / Published online: 08 November 2018
© Society for the Study of Inborn Errors of Metabolism (SSIEM) 2018

Abstract Ornithine transcarbamylase (OTC) deficiency is well known to cause severe neonatal hyperammonemia in males with absent enzyme activity. In families with large deletions of the X chromosome involving *OTC* and other contiguous genes, male infants appear to have an even more severe course. Notably, there are no published reports of these males surviving to liver transplant, even in cases where the diagnosis was known or suspected at birth. We describe two male newborns and their mother who all have a 1.5-Mb deletion of Xp11.4 encompassing the genes *TSPAN7*, *OTC*, and part of *RPGR*. The first child succumbed to his illness on his fourth day of life. His younger brother was diagnosed prenatally, and with early aggressive treatment, he survived the neonatal period. He suffered multiple life-threatening complications but stabilized and received a liver transplant at 7 months of age. This report demonstrates both the possibility of survival and the complications in caring for these patients.

Introduction

Ornithine transcarbamylase (OTC; OMIM 300461) is a proximal enzyme in the urea cycle which catalyzes the formation of citrulline from carbamoyl phosphate and ornithine. The gene *OTC* is located on the X chromosome at band Xp11.4. OTC deficiency (OMIM 311250) is the most common urea cycle disorder; in its classical form, it presents with severe neonatal hyperammonemia in affected males and has a mortality rate of 24% (Batshaw et al. 2014). This presentation typically occurs in males with null

mutations leading to absent enzyme activity in the liver (McCullough et al. 2000; Tuchman et al. 1989).

About 5–10% of cases of OTC deficiency are caused by deletions or complex rearrangements involving the *OTC* gene (Caldovic et al. 2015; Tuchman et al. 1998). Several families have been reported with large X chromosome deletions involving multiple genes, and the males described in these families seem to have a particularly poor prognosis, as described below in Table 1. Most affected males have died within days to weeks, and there are no published reports of these males receiving liver transplants. It has been proposed that the involvement of other genes in addition to *OTC* may complicate these patients' care (Balasubramaniam et al. 2010; Deardoff et al. 2008). The ratio of patients with deletions involving the *OTC* gene seems to be skewed heavily toward females, thought to be partially due to the diminished likelihood of survival in males (Shchelochkov et al. 2009).

Case 1

Patient 1 was born at 34 + 2 weeks' gestational age weighing 2,660 g. He was admitted to the neonatal intensive care unit (NICU) for prematurity following delivery and was started on standard total parenteral nutrition (TPN) and infant formula. On day 2 of life, he developed lethargy and seizures. He was loaded with phenobarbital and intubated. Labs were obtained which revealed an ammonia of 1,100 μmol/L. His IV fluids were immediately switched to dextrose 10% in water, and he was transferred to the children's hospital for further care. He was too hypotensive to safely initiate hemodialysis, so he was started on IV ammonia scavengers: sodium phenylacetate 250 mg/kg plus sodium benzoate 250 mg/kg and arginine 200 mg/kg, with one loading dose given over 2 h

Communicated by: Johannes Häberle

M. McPheron (✉) · M. Lah
Indiana University School of Medicine, Indianapolis, IN, USA
e-mail: mmcphero@iupui.edu

Table 1 Outcomes in male infants with OTC deficiency due to contiguous gene deletion syndromes

Reference	Deletion size, OMIM genes	Number of affected males	Positive family history?	Age at death
Gallant et al. (2015)	1.87-Mb deletion of *XK*, *CYBB*, *RPGR*, *OTC*, and *TSPAN7*	One	No	7 days old
Jain-Ghai et al. (2015)	0.74-Mb deletion of *RPGR*, *OTC*, and *TSPAN7*	One	Yes – older sister with known OTC deficiency	14 months old
Ono et al. (2010)	1-Mb deletion of *RPGR*, *OTC*, and *TSPAN7*	One	No	16 days old
Quental et al. (2009)	209-kb deletion of *OTC* and part of *TSPAN7*	One	No	Several days old
Deardoff et al. (2008)	3.9-Mb deletion of *XK*, *CYBB*, *RPGR*, and exons 1–8 of *OTC*	Two brothers	Yes – prenatal diagnosis made in second infant	5 days old (1st child) 12 weeks old (2nd child)
Arranz et al. (2007)	0.5-Mb deletion of *RPGR*, *OTC*, and *TSPAN7*	One	Yes – mother with known OTC deficiency	17 days old
Segues et al. (1995)	Both families had deletions of *CYBB*, *RPGR*, and *OTC*	Three: two brothers and one unrelated	Yes – one family had multiple male neonatal deaths	2 days old (both brothers) Several days old
Old et al. (1985)	Xp21 deletion on karyotype, spanning *NROB1* through *OTC*	One	No	36 h old

and a second dose given over the next 24 h. Labwork revealed glutamine 3,029 nmol/mL (reference range 316–1,020), citrulline 3 nmol/mL (reference range 9–38), and significantly elevated orotic acid and lactic acid in the urine. Despite treatment, his ammonia rose rapidly to 5,480 μmol/L on day 3 of life. Treatment was stopped, and he died on day 4 of life. Molecular analysis later revealed deletion of the entire *OTC* gene.

The patient's mother presented for a clinic visit 2 months later. She gave a personal history of sleepiness after eating meat and difficulty in school. Biochemical testing was significant for ammonia 42 μmol/L (reference range 11–35) and glutamine 1,060 nmol/mL (reference range 371–957). This information raised our suspicion that she may be a carrier of the deletion; however, confirmatory molecular testing was not done at that time due to insurance coverage. The maternal grandmother and great-grandmother both denied a history of symptoms, and there were no other males in the family who had died unexpectedly in infancy.

Genetic Testing

The patient's mother presented to prenatal diagnosis clinic when she was 25 weeks' pregnant with her second child. She opted for genetic testing via amniocentesis. Whole-genome array comparative genomic hybridization (CGH) was performed for both the fetus and the mother. The mother's report revealed a 1.5-Mb deletion at Xp11.4 and a 15-kb duplication at Xp22.33, reported as arr[hg19]

Xp22.33 (2,863,854–2,878,978)x3 and Xp11.4 (38,135,974–39,631,170)x1. The amniocentesis confirmed that the fetus was a male and carried both of these changes.

The Xp11.4 deletion encompasses *OTC* as well as three other genes: *TSPAN7* (transmembrane 4 superfamily member 2; OMIM 300096), *MID1IP1* (MID1 interacting protein 1; OMIM 300961), and part of *RPGR* (retinitis pigmentosa GTPase regulator; OMIM 312610). Both *RPGR* and *TSPAN7* have been linked to human diseases, whereas *MID1IP1* has not. Mutations in *RPGR* are a well-described cause of X-linked retinitis pigmentosa. Mutations in *TSPAN7*, also called *TM4SF2*, have been implicated in X-linked intellectual disability. The Xp22.33 duplication is classified as a variant of uncertain significance and contains part of the gene *ARSE* (arylsulfatase E; OMIM 300180). Mutations in *ARSE* can cause X-linked recessive chondrodysplasia punctata; the clinical significance of this duplication is unknown. The mother was monitored closely through the rest of her pregnancy and delivered at the academic medical center so that we could begin the baby's treatment immediately.

Case 2

Patient 2 was born at 38 + 3 weeks' gestational age weighing 3,283 g. Apgar scores were 8 and 9. He was immediately started on IV dextrose 10% in water, followed by IV ammonia scavengers started at 3 h of life. He was given a loading dose of sodium phenylacetate 250 mg/kg plus sodium benzoate 250 mg/kg and arginine 200 mg/kg given over 2 h, followed by a maintenance dose given over 24 h. His initial ammonia level at 3 h of life was 176 μmol/L and trended downward to a low of 67 μmol/L. He was started on continuous nasogastric tube feeds of Pro-Phree formula. The following day, his ammonia started to rise, and hemodialysis was started at 36 h of life. Ammonia peaked at 276 μmol/L before coming down to 35 μmol/L the following morning. On day 2, Cyclinex-1 formula was added to his feeds, providing 0.25 g/kg/day of protein in the form of essential amino acids. He was taken off of dialysis on day 4 of life and transitioned to enteral ammonia scavengers on day 6 of life: sodium phenylbutyrate 550 mg/kg/day and citrulline 200 mg/kg/day, each divided into four doses and given every 6 h. The amount of Cyclinex-1 in his feeds was increased, increasing protein intake to 0.5 g/kg/day on day 5 of life and to 1 g/kg/day on day 8 of life. His ammonia remained less than 50 μmol/L until reaching 1 g/kg/day of protein, at which time it peaked at 124 μmol/L and protein was temporarily decreased.

On day 13 of life, the baby developed sudden respiratory failure and went into cardiac arrest. He had had a normal exam and an ammonia level of 42 μmol/L earlier that morning. He received several rounds of CPR with epinephrine before his pulse returned. He was intubated and transferred to the pediatric intensive care unit (PICU) for postarrest care. His ammonia jumped to 778 μmol/L and lactate to >20 mmol/L. IV scavengers were restarted and the ammonia appropriately trended downward. He received infusions of epinephrine and norepinephrine for hypotension and cryoprecipitate and packed red blood cell transfusions for anemia and disseminated intravascular coagulopathy (DIC) and was started on a hypothermia protocol for neuroprotection. Blood cultures grew *Streptococcus mitis* in multiple bottles within 24 h, consistent with bacteremia.

Over the next few days, he slowly improved, and he was transferred out of the PICU for continued care when stable. He was transitioned back to enteral sodium phenylbutyrate and citrulline at the previously described dosing. A gastrostomy tube was placed, and he was kept on continuous drip feeds as we slowly increased his protein intake. Initially we increased the ratio of Cyclinex-1 to Pro-Phree formula to increase protein by 0.25 g/kg/day. Once he reached 1 g/kg/day of protein, we added ProSobee as a source of complete protein and continued to increase protein content by 0.25 g/kg/day until reaching 1.5 g/kg/day of protein, with total caloric goal within 110–120 kcal/kg/day. Ammonia levels remained less than 100 μmol/L during this time. His course continued to be otherwise complicated. He developed swelling and duskiness in the left foot and then the right

hand and was found to have thrombi in the left superficial femoral vein and the right jugular vein, both sites of previous central venous catheters, and was started on enoxaparin. He received several blood transfusions for anemia. He developed episodes of respiratory distress and vital sign changes consistent with sepsis around 4–5 weeks of age; blood, urine, and CSF cultures were all negative at that time. We continued to monitor him closely and determined that he was stable for discharge around 2 months of age: he was tolerating feeds, and his ammonia levels held steady around 50–60 μmol/L.

Over the next 5 months, he was followed closely in outpatient clinics. He saw either his pediatrician or his geneticist weekly for a weight check and an ammonia level. He had five admissions for ammonia levels above 100 μmol/L, typically related to viral infections. Two of these admissions required PICU-level care: the first due to an ammonia level of 282 μmol/L treated with IV scavengers and the second due to seizures, respiratory failure, and an ammonia level of 332 μmol/L treated with hemodialysis. During the other three admissions, he was treated conservatively with IV dextrose 10% and a brief reduction in protein intake, and he recovered quickly. Between hospitalizations, he tolerated 1.5 g/kg/day of protein in his feeds and maintained a normal weight. He was continued on enoxaparin by hematology, and workup revealed that he is heterozygous for the prothrombin 20210G>A mutation.

He was listed for liver transplant at 6 months of age, and he received a liver transplant at 7 months of age. The surgery was complicated by occlusive blood clots in the hepatic artery and portal vein which were removed in the operating room. He has been admitted several times posttransplant for respiratory illnesses and central line infections, though none have required PICU-level care. He continues to receive citrulline 200 mg/kg/day.

Patient 2 is currently 16 months old. He is behind in meeting developmental milestones but is making consistent progress. He is sitting unassisted and rolling over and working on putting pressure on his feet when held in a standing position. He transfers objects between his hands, waves, and drinks thickened liquids through a sippy cup. He is interactive, babbles, and says "hi" and "dada." His weight has never been below the second percentile. He appears to have some difficulty fixing visually as well as persistent nystagmus. Dilated eye exam does not show any retinal anomalies yet; electroretinography (ERG) may be considered in the future. His mother was advised to follow a protein-restricted diet and receives citrulline supplementation due to intermittently elevated glutamine levels, maximum of 1,150 nmol/mL (reference range 371–957). She has poor vision and endorses worsening vision at night. She is currently pregnant with an unaffected female.

Discussion

Deletions at Xp11.4 involving *OTC* and surrounding genes are expected to produce the most severe form of OTC deficiency. We saw this in our personal experience in taking care of this family, and this is reflected in prior literature which describes survival of weeks to months in most affected males. Males with absence of the entire gene are unable to make any amount of even truncated or minimally active enzyme. It has been previously proposed that the deletion of additional genes adds complexity (Deardoff et al. 2008), and we agree with this theory. *RPGR* is a protein involved in ciliary function and is expressed in the retina, respiratory tract epithelium, cochlea, and multiple other cell lines. Absence of this gene may have contributed to patient 2's multiple respiratory infections. *TSPAN7* is less well-described, and it is difficult to predict how this deletion is contributing to his developmental delays and hypotonia, especially in the setting of a previous cardiac arrest and multiple episodes of moderate hyperammonemia.

We attribute patient 2's survival, while his older brother had died, to prenatal diagnosis allowing for immediate treatment following delivery. His deletion was also smaller in size than some of the other male neonates who died, and notably did not contain *CYBB*, responsible for X-linked chronic granulomatous disease and thought to contribute to complications in other patients (Deardoff et al. 2008). Characterization of the deletion on cytogenetic testing allowed for us to have a realistic estimate of prognosis and to be prepared for a severe course. We recommend molecular testing in all those with a biochemical diagnosis of OTC deficiency and prenatal testing for at-risk fetuses for this reason. Another benefit of prenatal diagnosis is that it would allow for perinatal treatment. A recent paper describes the administration of IV sodium phenylacetate/ sodium benzoate and arginine to mothers during labor and delivery of male infants with severe defects in the *OTC* gene, and both infants had good neurodevelopmental outcomes (Wilnai et al. 2018). We agree that this is a reasonable approach in severe cases and may portend the best chance for survival.

Patient 2's long-term management was even more conservative than what we typically do for males with OTC deficiency. He was discharged from the NICU with both a gastrostomy tube and a tunneled central line for emergency management. Feeds were initially advanced slowly: we increased protein content by 0.25 g/kg/day, and we kept him on continuous rather than bolus feeds during that time to avoid giving him a large protein load at any one time. We also insisted that he was seen by a physician for an exam, weight check, and ammonia level test weekly. We admitted him for observation whenever his ammonia level rose above 100 µmol/L. He was ultimately listed for liver transplant by age 6 months. We would recommend a similar time frame in other males with severe neonatal disease to allow for the best chance of survival and a good neurocognitive outcome.

Acknowledgments We want to thank the patients' family for agreeing to participate in this report and for their amazing care of these young boys. We also acknowledge Dr. Bryan Hainline, Dr. Alyce Belonis, genetic counselors Katie Sapp and Kristyne Stone, and the rest of our care team who contributed greatly to the patients' clinical care.

Synopsis

OTC deficiency resulting from contiguous Xp11.4 gene deletion is typically fatal in male neonates, but with early and conservative management, survival to transplant is possible.

General Information

Author Contributions

- Molly McPheron: participated in patient care, researched pertinent literature, designed the outline of the report, wrote initial draft of the work, made corrections and revisions, approved final draft
- Melissa Lah: primary attending caring for the patients described, researched pertinent literature, involved in the design and planning of the paper, consulted during writing, revised the work, approved final draft

Conflicts of Interest

- Molly McPheron declares that she has no conflict of interest.
- Melissa Lah declares that she has no conflict of interest.

Funding

The authors did not use any sources of funding for this report.

Ethics Approval

This paper is exempt from IRB approval, as it is a case report and therefore does not qualify as human subject research.

Consent

The family gave their consent for us to write this case report. There is no identifying information included in this article. All procedures followed were in accordance with the ethical standards of the responsible committee on human experimentation (institutional and national) and with the Helsinki Declaration of 1975, as revised in 2000 (5). Informed consent was obtained from all patients for being included in the study. Proof that informed consent was obtained can be provided on request.

Animal Rights

This article does not contain any studies with animal subjects performed by any of the authors.

References

Arranz JA, Madrigal I, Ruidor E, Armengol L, Mila M (2007) Complete deletion of ornithine transcarbamylase gene confirmed by CGH array of X chromosome. J Inherit Metab Dis 30:813

Balasubramaniam S, Rudduck C, Bennetts B, Peters G, Wilcken B, Ellaway C (2010) Contiguous gene deletion syndrome in a female with ornithine transcarbamylase deficiency. Mol Genet Metab 99:34–41

Batshaw M, Tuchman M, Summar M, Seminara J (2014) A longitudinal study of urea cycle disorders. Mol Genet Metab 113:127–130

Caldovic L, Abdikarim I, Narain S, Tuchman M, Morizono H (2015) Genotype-phenotype correlations in ornithine transcarbamylase deficiency: a mutation update. J Genet Genomics 42(5):181–194

Deardoff MA, Gaddipati H, Kaplan P et al (2008) Complex management of a patient with a contiguous gene deletion involving ornithine transcarbamylase: a role for detailed molecular analysis in complex presentations of classical diseases. Mol Genet Metab 94:498–502

Gallant NM, Gui D, Lassman C et al (2015) Novel liver findings in ornithine transcarbamylase deficiency due to Xp11.4-p21.1 microdeletion. Gene 556:249–253

Jain-Ghai S, Skinner S, Hartley J, Fox S, Buhas D, Rockman-Greenberg C, Chan A (2015) Contiguous gene deletion of chromosome Xp in three families encompassing OTC, RPGR, and TSPAN 7 genes. J Rare Disord 1:1

McCullough BA, Yudkoff M, Batshaw ML, Wilson JM, Raper SE, Tuchman M (2000) Genotype spectrum of ornithine transcarbamylase deficiency: correlation with the clinical and biochemical phenotype. Am J Med Genet 93:313–319

Old JM, Purvis-Smith S, Wilcken B et al (1985) Prenatal exclusion of ornithine transcarbamylase deficiency by direct gene analysis. Lancet 325(8420):73–75

Ono M, Tsuda J, Mouri Y, Arai J, Arinami T, Noguchi E (2010) Contiguous Xp11.4 gene deletion leading to ornithine transcarbamylase deficiency detected by high-density single-nucleotide array. Clin Pediatr Endocrinol 19(2):25–30

Quental R, Azevedo L, Rubio V, Diogo L, Amoriam A (2009) Molecular mechanisms underlying large genomic deletions in ornithine transcarbamylase (OTC) gene. Clin Genet 75:457–464

Segues B, Rozet JM, Gilbert B et al (1995) Apparent segregation of null alleles ascribed to deletions of the ornithine transcarbamylase gene in congenital hyperammonemia. Prenat Diagn 15:757–761

Shchelochkov OA, Li FY, Geraghty MT et al (2009) High-frequency deletions and variable rearrangements at the ornithine transcarbamylase (OTC) locus by oligonucleotide array CGH. Mol Genet Metab 96:97–105

Tuchman M, Tsai MY, Holzknecht RA, Brusilow SW (1989) Carbamyl phosphate synthetase and ornithine transcarbamylase activities in enzyme-deficiency human liver measured by radiochromatography and correlated with outcome. Pediatr Res 26(1):77–82

Tuchman M, Morizono H, Rajagopal BS, Plante RJ, Allewell NM (1998) The biochemical and molecular spectrum of ornithine transcarbamylase deficiency. J Inherit Metab Dis 21(Suppl 1):40–58

Wilnai Y, Blumenfeld YJ, Cusmano K et al (2018) Prenatal treatment of ornithine transcarbamylase deficiency. Mol Genet Metab 123(3):297–300

JIMD Reports
DOI 10.1007/8904_2018_144

RESEARCH REPORT

The Unique Spectrum of Mutations in Patients with Hereditary Tyrosinemia Type 1 in Different Regions of the Russian Federation

G. V. Baydakova · T. A. Ivanova · S. V. Mikhaylova ·
D. Kh. Saydaeva · L. L. Dzhudinova ·
A. I. Akhlakova · A. I. Gamzatova · I. O. Bychkov ·
E. Yu. Zakharova

Received: 29 June 2018 / Revised: 29 August 2018 / Accepted: 17 September 2018 / Published online: 11 November 2018
© Society for the Study of Inborn Errors of Metabolism (SSIEM) 2018

Abstract *Background*: Hereditary tyrosinemia (HT1) is an autosomal recessive disorder characterized by impaired tyrosine catabolism because of fumarylacetoacetate hydrolase deficiency. HT1 is caused by homozygous or compound heterozygous mutations in the *FAH* gene. The HT1 frequency worldwide is 1:100,000–1:120,000 live births. The frequency of HT1 in the Russian Federation is unknown.

Aim: To estimate the spectrum of mutations in HT1 in several ethnic groups of the Russian Federation.

Materials and methods: From 2004 to 2017, 43 patients were diagnosed with HT1. The analysis of amino acids and succinylacetone was performed using NeoGram Amino Acids and Acylcarnitines Tandem Mass Spectrometry Kit and a Sciex QTrap 3200 quadrupole tandem mass spectrometer. Bi-directional DNA sequence analysis was performed on PCR products using an ABI Prism 3500.

Results: In the Russian Federation, the most common mutation associated with HT1 (32.5% of all mutant alleles) is c.1025C>T (p.Pro342Leu), which is typical for the Chechen ethnic group. Patients of the Yakut, the Buryat, and the Nenets origins had a homozygous mutation c.1090G>C (p.Glu364Gln). High frequency of these ethnicity-specific mutations is most likely due to the founder effect. In patients from Central Russia, the splicing site mutations c.554-1G>T and c.1062+5G>A were the most prevalent, which is similar to the data obtained in the Eastern and Central Europe countries.

Conclusion: There are ethnic specificities in the spectrum of mutations in the *FAH* gene in HT1. The Chechen Republic has one of the highest prevalence of HT1 in the world.

Communicated by: Piero Rinaldo, MD, PhD

G. V. Baydakova · T. A. Ivanova (✉) · I. O. Bychkov ·
E. Yu. Zakharova
Federal State Budgetary Scientific Institution "Research Center for Medical Genetics", Moscow, Russia
e-mail: breaking18@gmail.com

S. V. Mikhaylova
Russian Children's Clinical Hospital of the Ministry of Health of the Russian Federation, Moscow, Russia

D. Kh. Saydaeva · L. L. Dzhudinova
Perinatal Center, State Budgetary Institution Maternity Hospital, Grozny, The Chechen Republic, Russia

A. I. Akhlakova · A. I. Gamzatova
Republican Center for Medical Genetics, Makhachkala, The Republic of Dagestan, Russia

Introduction

Tyrosinemia type I (hepatorenal tyrosinemia (HT1) OMIM 276700) is an inherited disorder caused by deficiency of fumarylacetoacetate hydrolase (*FAH*, MIM 613871) which is the last enzyme of the tyrosine catabolic pathway. Enzyme deficiency leads to accumulation of toxic metabolites (succinylacetone and fumarylacetoacetate) that influence hepatocytes and cells of the proximal renal tubules, resulting in liver damage and disruption of tubular reabsorption of phosphates (Endo and Sun 2002; Novikov 2012).

The fumarylacetoacetate hydrolase gene (*FAH*) is located on chromosome 15 (locus 15q23-q25). To date, approximately 100 mutations have been found, and most of them are missense mutations (Bergeron et al. 2001).

HT1 is characterized by progressive liver disease and secondary renal tubular dysfunction leading to hypophosphatemic rickets. Two clinical forms of HT1 have been described: the acute form, which presents itself in the first months of life and is associated with acute liver failure, and the chronic form, which appears after the first year of age and leads to the development of hepatic failure or liver tumors (van Spronsen et al. 1994). The main biomarker used to detect the diagnosis of HT1 was an increase in succinylacetone (SA) in blood and urine.

Nitisinone (Orfadin®), also known as NTBC (2-(2-nitro-4-trifluoromethylbenzoyl)-1,3-cyclohexanedione), blocks the second step in the tyrosine degradation pathway and is successfully used for treatment of HT1. Therefore, early diagnosis of the disorder plays a crucial role in successful treatment (McKiernan 2006; Polyakova 2012).

Newborn screening for HT1 has been introduced in some countries and is based on detection of SA in the blood (Allard et al. 2004).

The aim of the study was to estimate the spectrum of mutations in HT1 and their frequencies in several ethnic groups belonging to different geographical regions of the Russian Federation.

Materials and Methods

Patients

From 2004 to 2017, 43 patients were diagnosed with HT1. The ethnic composition of the patients was as follows: 24 Russians, 13 Chechens, 1 Ingush, 2 Armenians, 1 Yakut, 1 Buryat, and 1 Nenets.

Metabolites

The analysis of amino acids, acylcarnitines, and succinylacetone was performed using NeoGram Amino Acids and Acylcarnitines Tandem Mass Spectrometry Kit (Perkin Elmer Life and Analytical Sciences, Wallac OY, Finland) and a Sciex QTrap 3200 (Sciex, USA) quadrupole tandem mass spectrometer operating based on the positive electrospray ionization technique. The concentrations of amino acids, acylcarnitines, and succinylacetone were calculated automatically using the internal standards and ChemoView software (Sciex, USA).

Molecular Genetics

Amplification of all the coding exons and their flanking regions FAH gene was performed by PCR on patient genomic DNA. Bi-directional DNA sequence analysis was performed on PCR products using an ABI Prism 3500 (Applied Biosystems). Primer sequences and protocol are available upon request.

To evaluate the frequency of the c.1025C>T (p. Pro342Leu) mutation, DNA extracted from dried blood spots of newborns from the Chechen Republic ($n = 2,215$) and the Republic of Dagestan ($n = 201$) were analyzed. Blood specimens (unidentified) were provided by the neonatal screening centers in Grozny and Makhachkala. The specimens were collected during 2016. PCR-RFLP analysis using MspI (C^CGG) restriction endonuclease (SibEnzyme, Russia) was developed for detection of the c.1025C>T (p.Pro342Leu) mutation. The Hardy-Weinberg equilibrium was used to calculate the frequency of the disorder: $p^2 + 2pq + q^2 = 1$. The confidence interval for frequencies was calculated by the Wilson method.

Results

In 43 patients from the Russian Federation, the diagnosis was made based on typical clinical presentation (hepatic impairment, rickets-like changes) as well as detection of specific HT1-related biomarkers, such as elevated blood and/or urine concentration of succinylacetone, tyrosine, and methionine. Biomarker concentrations in HT1 patients are presented in Table 1. In all patients, genetic testing was conducted to detect FAH gene mutations.

In our cohort of patients from different regions of the Russian Federation, 16 different mutations in different combinations were revealed; the most common mutations were c.554-1G>T, c.1062+5G>A, c.1025C>T (p.Pro342-Leu), and c.1090G>C (p.Glu364Gln). Clear ethnicity-related peculiarities were observed (Tables 2 and 3). The most frequent mutation in our cohort was c.1025C>T (p.Pro342Leu) (32.5% of mutant alleles).

Table 1 Biochemical changes observed in patients with tyrosinemia type 1

	Control[a]	Acute type[a]	Chronic type[a]
Tyrosine (blood), μM/L	81.7 ± 38.8 (3.1–322)	442 ± 136 (352.8–767)	327.1 ± 88.7 (234–618)
Methionine (blood), μM/L	26.8 ± 13.4 (3–198)	515.8 ± 318.8 (18.2–1,157)	45.1 ± 44.1 (11.3–171)
Succinylacetone (blood), μM/L	0.74 ± 0.3 (0.13–1.9)	32.1 ± 36.2 (5.27–85.2)	9.1 ± 5.9 (2.4–17.5)
Succinylacetone (urine), mM/M creatinine	Undetectable <2	167.3 ± 75.8 (75.4–283)	57.2 ± 33.3 (14–112)

[a] Mean ± deviation (minimum–maximum)

Table 2 Frequencies of the *FAH* gene mutations among patients with tyrosinemia type 1 from the Russian Federation

Mutation	Number of alleles	Frequency (%)
c.1025C>T (p.Pro342Leu)	28	32.5
c.554-1G>T (IVS6-1G>T)	20	23.3
c.1062+5G>A (IVS12 +5G>A)	8	9.3
c.1090G>C (p.Glu364Gln)	8	9.3
c.192G>T (p.Gln64His)	4	4.6
c.520C>T (p.Arg174Term)	2	2.3
c.782C>T (p.Pro261Leu)	2	2.3
c.497T>G (p.Val166Gly)	2	2.3
c.698A>T (p.Asp233Val)	1	1.2
c.2T>A (p.Met1Lys)	1	1.2
c.1056C>A (p.Ser352Arg)	1	1.2
c.455G>A (p.Trp152Term)	1	1.2
Variant of uncertain significance	8	9.3

Table 3 Frequencies of some mutations in the FAH gene in different ethnic groups

Ethnic group	Frequency of mutations (number of alleles)			
	c.554-1G>T	c.1062 +5G>A	c.1025C>T (p.Pro342Leu)	c.1090G>C (p.Glu364Gln)
Russians (n = 24)	**41.7 (20)**	**16.7 (8)**	0	0
Chechens (n = 13)	0	0	**100 (26)**	0
Armenians (n = 2)	0	0	0	0
Yakuts (n = 1)	0	0	0	**100 (2)**
Buryats (n = 1)	0	0	0	**100 (2)**
Nenets (n = 1)	0	0	0	**100 (2)**

Among 24 patients of Russian ethnic group, 20 alleles were identified c.554-1G>T, which is 41.7%; and 8 alleles were identified c.1062 +5G>A, which is 16.7% of the sample. 26 alleles c.1025C>T were found in 13 patients of the Chechen Republic, which is 100% of the sample. Yakuts, Buryats, and Nenets were found the same mutation in the homozygous state

Discussion

HT1 is a rare autosomal recessive genetic disorder. The HT1 worldwide frequency is approximately 1:100,000–1:120,000 live births (Mitchell et al. 2001). In some areas, the incidence of HT1 is noticeably higher. In Norway, Finland, and Tunisia, the frequency of HT1 is 1:74,800, 1:60,000, and

1:14,804, respectively (Bliksrud et al. 2012; St-Louis et al. 1994; Nasrallah et al. 2015). The highest prevalence of the disorder is observed in Canada (the Province of Quebec) near Saguenay-Lac Saint-Jean at 1:1,846 live births. Newborn screening has been conducted in the Province of Quebec since 1970. The most predominant mutation in this region is c.1062+5G>A (IVS12+5G>A), accounting for ~90% of all the disease-causing alleles. The HT1 carrier frequency in Quebec is 1:66, while in the region of Saguenay-Lac Saint-Jean, it is estimated to be 1:16–1:20 (De Braekeeler and Larochelle 1990).

In addition to the differences in incidence of the disorder, the distribution of mutations among ethnic groups has also been described. The most common mutation in patients from Northern Europe, Pakistan, Turkey, and the United States is a c.1062+5G>A (IVS12+5G>A) splicing mutation. Another splicing site mutation, c.554-1G>T, is prevalent in Central and Eastern Europe, and in Spain this mutation accounts for approximately 70% of all mutant alleles (Bergman et al. 1998). Some populations demonstrate predominance of certain unique mutations due to the founder effect. In the Finnish population, c.786G>A (p.Trp262X) represents ~88% of all reported HT1 alleles, and the major mutation in Ashkenazi Jews is c.782C>T (p.Pro261Leu) (St-Louis et al. 1994; Elpeleg et al. 2002). All patients from the Province of Quebec are homozygous for the splicing site mutation c.1062+5G>A (Elpeleg et al. 2002). In 19 HT1 patients in Norway, three new small deletions were found: c.615delT (p.Phe205LeufsX2), c.744delG (p.Pro249HisfsX55), and c.835delC (p. Gln279ArgfsX25) in 13.5%, 3.8%, and 1.9% of the alleles, respectively.

In our patients from Central Russia, the splicing site mutations c.554-1G>T and c.1062+5G>A were the most prevalent, which is similar to the data obtained in the Eastern and Central Europe countries (Table 3).

Clear ethnicity-related peculiarities were observed (Tables 2 and 3). The most frequent mutation in our cohort was c.1025C>T (p.Pro342Leu) (32.5% of mutant alleles). This homozygous mutation was identified in 14 patients, 13 of whom were ethnic Chechens (12 from the Chechen Republic and 1 from the Republic of Dagestan) and 1 was Ingush. This mutation has been previously described in the literature and in the Human Gene Mutation Database in a patient from Norway (HGMD CM940753) (heterozygous mutation). A functional analysis using fibroblast culture demonstrated a decrease in enzyme activity associated with this mutation (Rootwelt et al. 1994). Assessment of the mutation using standard software (PolyPhen-2, PROVEAN +SIFT, MutationTaster) shows highly probable pathogenicity of this substitution. According to ExAc, the frequency of this allele is 0.0000247/3, which also confirms its pathogenicity.

Based on the obtained results, it was suggested that the HT1 prevalence is higher in the Chechen Republic compared to other regions of the Russian Federation. The presence of the major mutation allows for analysis of the carrier frequency. 2,215 blood specimens collected from newborns in the Chechen Republic and 201 blood specimens collected from newborns in the Republic of Dagestan were analyzed. Thirty-five carriers of mutation c.1025C>T (p.Pro342Leu) were revealed in the Chechen population examined; no such mutation was found in the blood specimens obtained from newborns in the Republic of Dagestan. Thus, the frequency of the mutant allele p.Pro342Leu in the Chechen Republic was 0.0079 (95% confidence interval, 0.0045998 ± 0.01207), and the estimated frequency of HT1 (q^2) was 0.00006242 (95% confidence interval, $0.00002116 \pm 0.00014568$) or 1:16,020 (95% confidence interval, $1:6,864 \pm 1:47,263$). This frequency is one of the highest in the world. Since the Chechen population consists of local clans (taips), it is necessary to determine the taips of patients from the Chechen Republic to estimate the reason of prevalence of this mutation in the respective subpopulations (and to determine whether it is the result of the founder effect). Since the populations of the Chechens and the Ingush are genetically quite similar (Dibirova et al. 2010), it is reasonable to evaluate the frequency of the p.Pro342Leu mutation in the Ingush ethnic group.

Another interesting finding is the detection of a homozygous c.1090G>C (p.Glu364Gln) mutation in three patients (who were from the Yakut, Buryat, and Nenets ethnic groups). Maksimova et al. found that the carrier frequency of this heterozygous mutation among the Yakuts was 1%. These results suggest that the prevalence of HT1 in this region of the Russian Federation is also quite high and may be up to 1:10,000 live births (Maksimova et al. 2016).

In seven patients, undescribed variants in the heterozygous condition were identified (c.767C>A (p.Ala203Asp), c.772T>C (p.Phe205Ser), c.702G>T (p.Trp234Cys), c.803C>A (p.Ala268Asp), c.998A>C (p.His333Pro), c.706+3G>A (ivs8+3G>A), c.455+1G>A (ivs5 +1G>A)). Diagnosis of HT1 was confirmed by biochemical methods: succinylacetone in the urine ranged from 47 to 146 mM/M creatinine and in the blood ranged from 4 to 8 µM/L and tyrosine in the blood ranged from 113 to 618 µM/L. Functional diagnosis of confirmation of pathogenicity of the variants was not carried out. But assessment of the variants using standard software (PolyPhen-2, PROVEAN+SIFT, MutationTaster) shows highly probable pathogenicity of these substitutions. It should be noted that the variant c.772T>C (p.Phe205Ser) met twice by patients of the Chuvash Republic.

Common pseudodeficiency allele c.1021C>T (p. Arg341Trp) was not detected in patients with HT1. Frequency of this allele was about 3% in the control sample.

Conclusion

Evaluation of the spectrum of mutations in the *FAH* gene in hereditary tyrosinemia type 1 (HT1) in different populations of the Russian Federation demonstrated ethnic specificity of some mutations. The mutation c.1025C>T (Pro342Leu), which is common for the Chechens, was found to be the most common (32.5%) among mutations leading to this disorder. The estimated prevalence of HT1 in this population, 1:16,020, is one of the highest in the world.

We identify mutation c.1090G>C (p.Glu364Gln), in HT1 patients representing the nations of the peoples of Northern-Eastern Russia, including the Yakuts, the Buryats, and the Nenets. The estimated prevalence of HT1 in the Yakuts may be 1:10,000 live births, which is also quite high.

The obtained data indicate the need for introduction of HT1 newborn screening to the National program in the Chechen Republic and probably in Yakutia.

The authors declare that there is no conflict of interest.

Compliance with Ethics Guidelines

Galina Baydakova, Tatiana Ivanova, Svetlana Mikhaylova, Djamila Saydaeva, Laura Dzhudinova, Ayashat Akhlakova, Amina Gamzatova, Igor Bychkov, and Ekaterina Zakharova declare that they have no conflict of interest.

This study was partially granted by SOBI.

All procedures followed were in accordance with the ethical standards of the responsible committee on human experimentation (institutional and national) and with the Helsinki Declaration of 1975, as revised in 2000 (5). Informed consent was obtained from all patients for being included in the study.

This article does not contain any studies with human or animal subjects performed by the any of the authors.

Baydakova G. V. performed the analysis of amino acids and succinylacetone in spots of dried blood, conducted DNA diagnostics to detect mutations in the FAH gene, calculated the frequency of the disorder, and calculated the confidence interval for frequencies.

Ivanova T. A. performed the analysis of amino acids and succinylacetone in spots of dried blood and conducted DNA diagnostics to detect mutations in the FAH gene.

Mikhaylova S. V. carried out a sample of patients on the territory of the Russian Federation and selection and search of articles and literature.

Saydaeva D. Kh. and Dzhudinova L. L. carried out a sample of patients on the territory of the Chechen Republic and selection and search of articles and literature.

Akhlakova A. I. and Gamzatova A. I. carried out a sample of patients on the territory of the Republic of Dagestan and selection and search of articles and literature.

Bychkov I. O. conducted DNA diagnostics to detect mutations in the FAH gene.

Zakharova E. Yu is the guarantor of the research.

Competing Interests

None declared.

References

Allard P, Grenier A, Korson MS, Zytkovicz TH (2004) Newborn screening for hepatorenal tyrosinemia by tandem mass spectrometry: analysis of succinylacetone extracted from dried blood spots. Clin Biochem 37(11):1010–1015

Bergeron A, D'Astous M, Timm DE, Tanguay RM (2001) Structural and functional analysis of missense mutations in fumarylacetoacetate hydrolase, the gene deficient in hereditary tyrosinemia type 1. J Biol Chem 276:15225–15231

Bergman AJ, van den Berg IE, Brink W et al (1998) Spectrum of mutations in the fumarylacetoacetate hydrolase gene of tyrosinemia type 1 patients in northwestern Europe and Mediterranean countries. Hum Mutat 12(1):19–26

Bliksrud YT, Brodtkorb E, Backe PH et al (2012) Hereditary tyrosinaemia type I in Norway: incidence and three novel small deletions in the fumarylacetoacetase gene. Scand J Clin Lab Invest 72(5):369–373

De Braekeeler M, Larochelle J (1990) Genetic epidemiology of hereditary tyrosinemia in Quebec and the Saguenay-Lac-St-Jean. Am J Hum Genet 47(2):302–307

Dibirova KD, Balanovskaya EV, Kuznetzova MA et al (2010) Genetic topography of the Caucasus: four linguistic-geographical regions as indicated by data on chromosome Y polymorphism. Med Genet 10:10–14 (in Russian)

Elpeleg ON, Shaag A, Holme E et al (2002) Mutation analysis of the FAH gene in Israeli patients with tyrosinemia type I. Hum Mutat 19(1):80–81

Endo F, Sun MS (2002) Tyrosinaemia type I and apoptosis of hepatocytes and renal tubular cells. J Inherit Metab Dis 25:227–234

Maksimova NR, Gurinova EE, Sukhomyasova AL et al (2016) A novel homozygous mutation causing hereditary tyrosinemia type I in Yakut patient in Russia: case report. Wiad Lek 69(2 Pt 2):295–298

McKiernan PJ (2006) Nitisinone in the treatment of hereditary tyrosinaemia type 1. Drugs 66(6):743–750

Mitchell GA, Grompe M, Lambert M, Tanguay RM (2001) Hypertyrosinemia. In: Scriver CR, Beaudet AL, Sly WS, Valle D (eds) The metabolic and molecular bases of inherited disease. McGraw Hill, New York, pp 1777–1806

Nasrallah F, Hammami MB, Ben Rhouma H et al (2015) Clinical and biochemical profile of tyrosinemia type 1 in Tunisia. Clin Lab 61(5–6):487–492

Novikov PV (2012) Tyrosinemia type I: clinical signs, diagnosis and treatment. Russ Bull Perinatol Pediatr S3:1–27 (in Russian)

Polyakova SI (2012) Effectiveness of nitisinone therapy for hereditary tyrosinemia type I. Russ Pediatr J 6:59–60 (in Russian)

Rootwelt H, Chou J, Gahl WA, Berger R, Coşkun T, Brodtkorb E, Kvittingen EA (1994) Two missense mutations causing tyrosinemia type 1 with presence and absence of immunoreactive fumarylacetoacetase. Hum Genet 93(6):615–619

St-Louis M, Leclerc B, Laine J et al (1994) Identification of a stop mutation in five Finnish patients suffering from hereditary tyrosinemia type I. Hum Mol Genet 3(1):69–72

van Spronsen FJ, Thomasse Y, Smit GP, Leonard JV et al (1994) Hereditary tyrosinemia type I: a new clinical classification with difference in prognosis on dietary treatment. Hepatology 20:1187–1191

JIMD Reports
DOI 10.1007/8904_2018_146

RESEARCH REPORT

Elevated Lyso-Gb3 Suggests the R118C GLA Mutation Is a Pathological Fabry Variant

Andrew Talbot · Kathy Nicholls

Received: 22 July 2018 / Revised: 13 October 2018 / Accepted: 08 November 2018 / Published online: 20 December 2018
© Society for the Study of Inborn Errors of Metabolism (SSIEM) 2018

Abstract *Background*: Fabry disease (FD), an X-linked lysosomal storage disease, results from an α-galactosidase A deficiency and altered sphingolipid metabolism. An accumulation of globotriaosylsphingosine (lyso-Gb3) likely triggers the pathological cascade leading to disease phenotype. The pathogenic significance of several Fabry mutations including the R118C α-galactosidase (GLA) gene variant has been disputed. We describe three members of the same family with the R118C variant, each having documented clinical signs of FD, low residual enzyme levels, and an elevated lyso-Gb3 in one heterozygote.

Determining the clinical significance of each GLA gene variant remains an ongoing challenge, with potential for inadequate treatment if the diagnosis of FD is missed. Elevated lyso-Gb3 has been shown to be the most reliable noninvasive marker of clinically relevant GLA variants. While the R118C variant will likely lead to a milder phenotype, additional genetic, epigenetic, and environmental factors can ameliorate or exacerbate the expression and impact on the resultant phenotype and associated complications. Patients affected with this variant warrant closer review and better management of disease risk factors.

Abbreviations

αGal	Alpha-galactosidase A
FD	Fabry disease
Gb3	Globotriaosylceramide
GLA	Gene encoding α-galactosidase
Lyso Gb3	Globotriaosylsphingosine

Introduction

Fabry disease (FD) (OMIM 301500) is an X-linked lysosomal storage disease with reduced α-galactosidase A (αGal) activity (Desnick et al. 1973) and disrupted glycosphingolipid homeostasis resulting from mutations in the α-galactosidase (GLA) gene. Intracellular accumulation of the glycosphingolipid globotriaosylceramide (Gb3) triggers inflammation, hypertrophy, and fibrosis and causes widespread organ injury (von Scheidt et al. 1991). More than 700 GLA gene variants have been reported (Smid et al. 2015), 60% being mis-sense mutations, leading to a significant heterogeneity in phenotype, even within families carrying the same variant. Accurate and reliable diagnosis of FD and the potential phenotype–genotype relationship is extremely important in patient management.

In classical FD, patients have very low or no residual αGal activity, with resultant life-threatening end-organ injury including progressive hypertrophic cardiomyopathy, renal impairment, and cerebrovascular disease including strokes (Mehta et al. 2009). Another group of patients have delayed or attenuated forms of FD, presenting clinically with single organ involvement, often cardiac, or with milder phenotypes (Desnick et al. 2003). These variants tend to be associated with higher residual but still subnormal αGal activity. A third group of GLA variants, including D313Y and S126G, have been described as non-organ affecting (Linthorst et al. 2010;

Communicated by: Martina Huemer

A. Talbot (✉) · K. Nicholls
Department of Nephrology, Royal Melbourne Hospital, Parkville, VIC, Australia
e-mail: andrew.talbot@mh.org.au

K. Nicholls
Department of Medicine, University of Melbourne, Parkville, VIC, Australia

Houge et al. 2011). These variants have been reported to have residual enzyme levels above that likely to cause disease (Schiffmann et al. 2016). The GLA variant R118C has previously been included in this nonpathogenic group based on the absence of end-organ pathology in a large Portuguese family (Ferreira et al. 2015).

The deacylated form of globotriaosylsphingosine (lyso-Gb3) has been suggested as a biomarker of disease. Lyso-Gb3 accumulates in vasoendothelial cells and has been detected at a high level in plasma (Aerts et al. 2008). It correlates with left ventricular hypertrophy (Aerts et al. 2008; Rombach et al. 2010) and has been associated with the development of cerebrovascular accidents and white matter lesions (Rombach et al. 2010). Elevated lyso-Gb3 has therefore been recommended as an accurate determinant and noninvasive indication of clinically significant Fabry disease (Nowak et al. 2017). We therefore challenge the assertion that R118C is nonpathogenic, based on our clinical and biochemical findings in three family members with this mutation.

Methods

All samples were processed by the South Australian Pathology Service, the National referral Laboratory for Metabolic disease analysis, a Nationally Accredited facility. Genetic determination of Fabry sequence variants was performed on blood EDTA samples with restriction enzyme analysis. Alpha-Galctosidase activity was measured in dried blood spot samples. Lyso Gb3 was assayed by LC/MS (Talbot et al. 2017).

Peripheral neuropathy was determined by bedside examination including thermal discrimination testing.

Case Report

A 25-year-old heterozygous female with a family history of cardiovascular disease was identified as carrying the R118C GLA gene variant of FD through screening for familial cardiomyopathy. Plasma αGal activity was 1.5 nmol/h/mL (Normal 2.0–6.9 nmol/h/mL) on dried blood spot and lyso-Gb3 was 5 pmol/mL (Normal <5 pmol/mL). Clinical features included peripheral neuropathy, with temperature analgesia in hands and feet, hypohidrosis, and mild septal hypertrophy, but no proteinuria or cerebrovascular disease (see Table 1). In the absence of altered renal or cardiac function there were no indications for cardiac or renal biopsies. She has not to date been referred for enzyme replacement therapy.

The father of the index case, a 60-year-old homozygous male with hypertension, had reduced αGAL activity at

1.4 nmol/h/mL on dried blood spot, but no elevation in lyso-Gb3. Clinical signs included mild concentric left ventricular hypertrophy, cerebrovascular disease manifesting as white matter lesions, hypohidrosis, and peripheral neuropathy with temperature analgesia in hands and feet. In the absence of altered renal or significant cardiac dysfunction there were no indications for cardiac or renal biopsies. He has not been referred for enzyme replacement therapy at this point.

The sister of the index case, a 28-year-old heterozygous female, had αGal activity at the lower level of normal at 2.0 nmol/h/mL (Normal 2.0–6.9 nmol/h/mL) on dried blood spot, and no elevation in lyso-Gb3. Clinically she had hypohidrosis, temperature analgesia to hands and feet, and gastrointestinal symptoms. Of note she had a long cardiac history with symptomatic heart block requiring a pacemaker and cardiomegaly. A cardiac biopsy performed several years earlier showed occasional small and single lamellar bodies consistent with early Fabry disease. These pathological Fabry findings however were out of keeping with the severity of her cardiac disease suggesting a second pathology exacerbating her presentation.

Discussion

In classical FD phenotypes, diagnosis is established by low αGal levels, most reliably in males, and increased lyso-Gb3 in tissues or plasma (Schiffmann et al. 2016; Desnick et al. 1973). The pathological GLA mutation is then identified by genetic testing. Lyso-Gb3 has been confirmed as a biochemical marker in cases of uncertain diagnosis (Aerts et al. 2008; Nowak et al. 2017). We present clear evidence of the potential pathogenicity of the R118C GLA gene variant. Within our R118C family, three members had clinical phenotype of hypohidrosis, temperature analgesia, and reduced αGal levels, while an elevated plasma lyso-Gb3 was present in one heterozygote, and a cardiac biopsy showed early Fabry related changes in another. While disease severity is mild in this family, a diagnosis of mild but clinically significant FD has been established. This diagnosis has the potential to dramatically alter patient management, including the necessity for close monitoring and provision for prophylactic therapy against disease complications.

This family highlights both the difficulties of definitive causality of some GLA mutations in Fabry disease and the need for accurate biomarkers. Clinical signs were supportive of the diagnosis in each patient but have been debated in the literature. Definitive tissue morphology was limited to a single cardiac biopsy with only early Fabry changes. Indeed it is likely that a second pathology like a viral associated cardiomyopathy exacerbated this patient's presentation.

Table 1 Baseline clinical features of relatives with the R118C GLA mutation

	Patient 1	Patient 2	Patient 3
Age	25	60	28
Gender	Female	Male	Female
α-galactosidase A (normal 2.0–6.9 nmol/h/mL)	1.5	1.4	2.0
Lyso Gb3 (pmol/mL)	5	Not elevated	Not elevated
BMI kg/m^2	24.9	32.5	39
Symptoms			
Hypohidrosis	Yes	Anhidrosis	Yes
Angiokeratoma	Nil	Scattered	Nil
Neuropathic pain	Nil	Nil	Moderate
Gastrointestinal	Nil	Nil	Diarrhoea
Dyspnoea	Nil	Nil	NYHA 2
Cardiac			
ECG	NAD	LVH	Paced/bradycardia
IVSD (mm)	11	11	8
PWT (mm)	7	11	9
E/Ea	–	11	–
Renal			
eGFR (MDRD)	112	129	83
Proteinuria (g/24 h)	0.12	0.18	0.13
Serum creatinine	57	56	72
Neurological			
MRI brain			
WML	Nil	Mild	–
CVA	Nil	Nil	–
Ectasia	Nil	Mild	–
Neuropathy	Temperature analgesia	Temperature analgesia	Temperature analgesia

However, left ventricular hypertrophy has been described previously in a patient with this R118C mutation (Caetano et al. 2014). Recently Lyso-Gb3 has become established as a noninvasive maker for the presence of Fabry disease (Nowak et al. 2017). Where serum lyso-Gb3 is detected it serves as a marker of tissue involvement but its absence does not preclude tissue injury. Given that there has been debate in the literature about the cut-off of pathological lyso-Gb3 levels we have previously published a lyso-Gb3 assay (Talbot et al. 2017) with high cut-off of 5 pmol/mL such that there are no false positive results. However, aside from establishing the diagnosis, the correlation between specific disease mutations and lyso-Gb3 levels (Lukas et al. 2013) has not yet been proven, especially in females. Indeed lyso-Gb3 is not elevated in the late-onset M296I mutation (Mitobe et al. 2012) and 19% of females with the IVS4 + 914G>A mutation have lyso Gb3 within the normal range (Liao et al. 2013). Other studies however

suggest that lyso-Gb3 levels can differentiate clinically relevant Fabry mutations (Lukas et al. 2013; Niemann et al. 2014; Nowak et al. 2017) and can separate high-risk affected females with the late-onset IVS4 + 914G>A mutation from unaffected controls (Liao et al. 2013). Furthermore there is currently no plasma lysoGb3 concentration that can predict either the absence or the presence of end-organ damage.

As in many diseases multiple additional genetic and epigenetic factors are likely to ameliorate or exacerbate the impact of each Fabry mutation, and hence underlie the significant heterogeneity of disease. For example, in FD patients with the p.A143T GLA mutation, the 10C>T polymorphism in the 5′ untranslated region of GLA has been shown to reduce alpha-galactosidase activity (Desnick et al. 2015). This could partially explain the pathogenic variability seen in this mutation. Whether a similar polymorphism can explain the variability in the R118C mutation has not been shown. In any case family members with this mutation require ongoing assessment and end-organ investigation.

Acknowledgments   The authors thank Elizabeth Centra and Donna North for sample preparation and testing of all Fabry patients.

Take Home Message

The Fabry R118C GLA mutation may cause clinically significant disease with reduced α galactosidase level and requires ongoing patient follow-up.

Compliance with Ethics Guidelines

Details of Contributions of Individual Authors

Andrew Talbot was responsible for data interpretation and original manuscript preparation.

Kathy Nicholls was involved in data interpretation and original manuscript preparation.

Conflict of Interest

Nil direct.

Andrew Talbot has received research support, speaker honoraria, and travel assistance from Shire Corporation and Sanofi Corporation, speaker honoraria and travel assistance from Dainippon Sumitomo Pharma Co, and research support from Amicus Therapeutics and Protalix Biotherapeutics.

Kathy Nicholls has received research support, speaker honoraria, and travel assistance from Shire Corporation and Sanofi Corporation and research support from Amicus Therapeutics and Protalix Biotherapeutics.

Informed Consent

All procedures followed were in accordance with the ethical standards of the responsible committee on human experimentation (institutional and national) and with the Helsinki Declaration of 1975, as revised in 2000(5). Informed consent was obtained from all patients for data analysis of results included in the study.

References

Aerts JM, Groener JE, Kuiper S et al (2008) Elevated globotriaosylceramide is a hallmark of Fabry disease. Proc Natl Acad Sci U S A 105(8):2812–2817

Caetano F, Botelho A, Mota P, Silva J, Leitão Margues A (2014) Fabry disease presenting as apical left ventricular hypertrophy in a patient carrying the missense mutation R118C. Rev Port Cardiol 33(3):183.e1–183.e5

Desnick RJ, Allen KY, Desnick SJ, Raman MK, Bernlohr RW, Krivit W (1973) Fabry's disease: enzymatic diagnosis of hemizygotes and heterozygotes. Alpha-galactosidase activities in plasma, serum, urine and leukocytes. J Lab Clin Med 81:157–171

Desnick RJ, Brady R, Barranger J et al (2003) Fabry disease, an under-recognized multisystemic disorder: expert recommendations for diagnosis, management, and enzyme replacement therapy. Ann Intern Med 138:338–346

Desnick RJ, Doheny D, Chen B et al (2015) Fabry disease: the α-galactosidase A (GLA) c.427G>A (A143T) mutation, effect of the 5'-10C>T polymorphism. Mol Genet Metab 114:S11–S130

Ferreira S, Ortiz O, Germain DP et al (2015) The alpha-galactosidase A p.Arg118Cys variant does not cause a Fabry disease phenotype: data from individual patients and family studies. Mol Genet Metab 114:248–258

Houge G, Tondel C, Kaarboe O, Hirth A, Bostad L, Svarstad E (2011) Fabry or not Fabry – a question of ascertainment. Eur J Hum Genet 19:1111

Linthorst GE, Bouwman MG, Wijburg FA, Aerts JM, Poorthuis BJ, Hollak CE (2010) Screening for Fabry disease in high-risk populations: a systematic review. J Med Genet 47:217–222

Liao H-C, Huang Y-H, Kao S-M et al (2013) Plasma globotriaosylsphingosine (lysoGb3) could be a biomarker for Fabry disease with a Chinese hotspot late-onset mutation (IVS4 + 919G>A). Clin Chim Acta 426:114–120

Lukas J, Giese A, Markoff A et al (2013) Functional characterisation of alpha-galactosidase a mutations as a basis for a new classification system in Fabry disease. PLOS Genet 9(8): e1003632

Mehta A, Clarke JTR, Giugliani R, Elliott P, Linhart A, Beck M, Sunder-Plassmann, on behalf of the FOS Investigators (2009) Natural course of Fabry disease: changing pattern of causes of death in FOS – Fabry Outcome Survey. J Med Genet 46:548–552

Mitobe S, Togawa T, Tsukimara T et al (2012) Mutant α galactosidase A with M296I dose not cause elevation of the plasma globotriaosylsphingosine level. Mol Genet Metab 104:623–626

Niemann M, Rolfs A, Störk S et al (2014) Gene mutations versus clinical relevant phenotypes. Lyso-Gb3 defines Fabry disease. Circ Cardiovasc Genet 7:8–16

Nowak A, Mechtler TP, Desnick RJ, Kasper DC (2017) Plasma LysoGb3: a useful biomarker for the diagnosis and treatment of Fabry disease heterozygotes. Mol Genet Metab 120:57–61

Rombach SM, Dekker N, Bouwman MG et al (2010) Plasma globotriaosylsphingosine: diagnostic value and relation to clinical manifestations of Fabry disease. Biochim Biophys Acta 1802:741–748

Schiffmann R, Fuller M, Clarke LA, Aerts JM (2016) Is it Fabry's disease? Genet Med 18(12):1181–1185

Smid BE, van der Tol L, Biegstraaten M et al (2015) Plasma globotriaosylsphingosine in relations to phenotypes of Fabry disease. J Med Genet 52:262–268

Talbot A, Nicholls K, Fletcher J, Fuller M (2017) A simple method for quantification of plasma globotriaosylsphingosine: utility for Fabry disease. Mol Genet Metab 122:121–125

von Scheidt W, Eng CM, Fitzmaurice TF et al (1991) An atypical variant of Fabry's disease with manifestations confined to the myocardium. N Engl J Med 324:395–399

JIMD Reports
DOI 10.1007/8904_2018_148

RESEARCH REPORT

Glycogen Storage Disease Type IV: A Rare Cause for Neuromuscular Disorders or Often Missed?

Imre F. Schene · Christoph G. Korenke ·
Hidde H. Huidekoper · Ludo van der Pol ·
Dennis Dooijes · Johannes M. P. J. Breur ·
Saskia Biskup · Sabine A. Fuchs · Gepke Visser

Received: 24 April 2018 / Revised: 14 September 2018 / Accepted: 18 October 2018 / Published online: 20 December 2018
© Society for the Study of Inborn Errors of Metabolism (SSIEM) 2018

Abstract Advancements in genetic testing now allow early identification of previously unresolved neuromuscular phenotypes. To illustrate this, we here present diagnoses of glycogen storage disease IV (GSD IV) in two patients with hypotonia and delayed development of gross motor skills. Patient 1 was diagnosed with congenital myopathy based on a muscle biopsy at the age of 6 years. The genetic cause of his disorder (two compound heterozygous mis-sense mutations in *GBE1* (c.[760A>G] p.[Thr254Ala] and c.[1063C>T] p.[Arg355Cys])), however, was only identified at the age of 17, after panel sequencing of 314 genes associated with neuromuscular disorders. Thanks to the availability of next-generation sequencing, patient 2 was diagnosed before the age of 2 with two compound heterozygous mutations in *GBE1* (c.[691+2T>C] (splice donor variant) and the same c.[760A>G] p.[Thr254Ala] mutation as patient 1). GSD IV is an autosomal recessive metabolic disorder with a broad and expanding clinical spectrum, which hampers targeted diagnostics. The current cases illustrate the value of novel genetic testing for rare genetic disorders with neuromuscular phenotypes, especially in case of clinical heterogeneity. We argue that genetic testing by gene panels or whole exome sequencing should be considered early in the diagnostic procedure of unresolved neuromuscular disorders.

Communicated by: Terry G. J. Derks

Electronic supplementary material: The online version of this chapter (https://doi.org/10.1007/8904_2018_148) contains supplementary material, which is available to authorized users.

I. F. Schene · S. A. Fuchs · G. Visser (✉)
Department of Metabolic Diseases, Wilhelmina Children's Hospital, University Medical Centre Utrecht, Utrecht, The Netherlands
e-mail: G.Visser-4@umcutrecht.nl

C. G. Korenke
Department of Neuropediatrics, Children's Hospital Klinikum Oldenburg, Oldenburg, Germany

H. H. Huidekoper
Department of Pediatrics, Center for Lysosomal and Metabolic Diseases, Erasmus Medical Center, Rotterdam, The Netherlands

L. van der Pol
Department of Neurology, University Medical Centre Utrecht, Utrecht, The Netherlands

D. Dooijes
Department of Medical Genetics, University Medical Center Utrecht, Utrecht, The Netherlands

J. M. P. J. Breur
Department of Pediatric Cardiology, Wilhelmina Children's Hospital, University Medical Centre Utrecht, Utrecht, The Netherlands

S. Biskup
CeGaT GmbH and Praxis für Humangenetik Tübingen, Tübingen, Germany
e-mail: Saskia.Biskup@humangenetik-tuebingen.de

Introduction

Rapidly evolving genetic diagnostic procedures provide a powerful tool to unravel the disease cause in pediatric patients with a suspected genetic disorder. Specifically, this advancement allows identification of mild or atypical phenotypes of rare Mendelian diseases (Choi et al. 2009). Our recent identification of glycogen storage disease type IV (GSD IV) [OMIM 232500] in two patients with congenital myopathy serves as a good example.

GSD IV is an autosomal recessive inborn error of metabolism caused by mutations in the gene-encoding glycogen-branching enzyme (GBE1, EC 2.4.1.18). This enzyme is critical for the production of normal glycogen. Reduced activity causes linear glycogen with long chains of

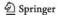

glucose and infrequent branch points. The resulting amylo-pectin-like polysaccharide (polyglucosan) accumulates in all tissues, most notably in liver and muscle. The GSD IV phenotype represents a heterogeneous continuum of disease that ranges from perinatal, early fatal neuromuscular disease, to severe isolated hepatopathy requiring liver transplantation, to mild myopathy (Moses and Parvari 2002; Magoulas and El-Hattab 2013). Adult polyglucosan body disease (APBD), characterized by progressive dys-function of central and peripheral nervous system in adulthood, is caused by mutations in the same gene (Klein 2013).

The two patients described here both presented with hypotonia, delayed development of gross motor skills, and mild failure to thrive. The "diagnostic odyssey" of patient 1 was long and only ended after the advent of next-generation sequencing when he was aged 17. In contrast, the genetic defect in patient 2 was identified within the first 2 years of life, illustrating the advancement of genetic diagnostics in patients with unresolved neuromuscular phenotypes.

Case Report

Case Description 1

After a normal pregnancy and delivery, patient 1 (male) was born to nonconsanguineous parents and presented with late development of gross motor skills. Neck holding, crawling, and standing were all delayed by several months. Fine motor, cognitive, and verbal development were normal. Clinically, he showed weakness and hypotrophy of all large muscles. No sensory, pyramidal, or cerebellar deficits were present and motor nerve conduction was normal. Creatine

kinase was always in the normal range (80–160 U/L) and no abnormalities in the DMPK gene were found. At age 6 years, a muscle biopsy showed mild fiber-type dispropor-tion without any signs pointing towards a more specific disorder, such as (polyglucosan) inclusion bodies. At 7 years of age, his growth was stunted with length 114 cm (−2 SD) and weight-to-length ratio 16 kg/114 cm (−2.4 SD). At age 8, mild hepatomegaly was noticed (1–2 cm below costal margin), liver transaminases were mildly increased (ALP max 219 U/L, AST max 116 U/L, and ALT max 73 U/L), and prolonged overnight fasting caused symptoms compat-ible with hypoglycemia. Indeed, a regular fasting test showed diminished fasting tolerance (blood glucose <3.0 mmol/L after 15 h).

To further investigate the nature of this intolerance, a fasting test with use of stable isotopes was performed at age 9 in which blood glucose was 3.4 mmol/L after 16 h of fasting (Fig. 1a). Endogenous glucose production (EGP) remained within the normal range, but the fractional glycogenolysis (GGL) was lower than the reported fractional GGL for healthy controls (Fig. 1b, also see Supplementary Material). Lacking an exact, genetic expla-nation for this glycogenolytic deficiency, a functional diet approach was started that aimed at preventing catabolism and consisted of three large meals, frequent smaller meals, and an evening dose of raw cornstarch (40 g). This diet led to compensatory growth, normalization of gross motor skills, and improvement of exercise tolerance. He was able to cycle 22 km each day, but still experienced exhaustion at the end of the day. At age 17, another fasting test was performed to assess the safety of extended fasting given his intention to live independently in student housing. During the fasting test glucose concentration now remained above

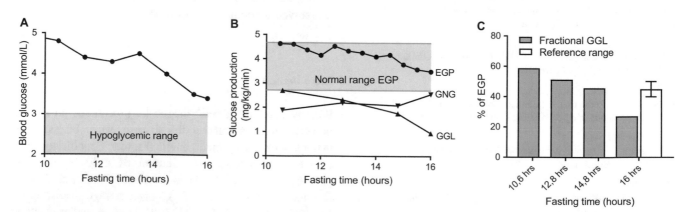

Fig. 1 Glucose kinetics during a fasting test in patient 1, including (**a**) plasma glucose concentrations, (**b**) endogenous glucose production (EGP; circle), glycogenolysis (GGL; triangle), and gluconeogenesis (GNG; inverted triangle), and (**c**) fractional glycogenolysis in relation to the fasting time

4.5 mmol/L after 17 h of fasting. This initiated a new diagnostic work-up, including next generations sequencing which by then had become available and affordable.

Genetic Evaluation

Genetic investigation of 314 genes associated with neuromuscular disorders revealed two compound heterozygous missense mutations in the *GBE1* gene (NM_00158.3): c.[760A>G] p.[Thr254Ala] (previously reported, Said et al. 2016) and c.[1063C>T] p.[Arg355Cys] (previously unreported). Three pathogenicity prediction algorithms (PolyPhen-2: both damaging, MutationAssesor: T253A = medium impact, R355C = high impact, MutationTaster2: both disease causing) predicted T254A to have medium impact and R355C to have high impact on protein function. The activity of GBE1 in white blood cells was severely impaired compared to reference values. The muscle biopsy taken at age 6 was re-examined, but no polyglucosan bodies, which could have been diagnostic for GSD IV, could be identified.

Radiographic Evaluation

To further investigate the muscular phenotype, we performed a whole body MRI scan at age 17. This scan showed bilateral atrophy of the gluteus maximus muscle and mild atrophy of the semimembranosus muscle (Fig. 2). The muscle MRIs showed no edema, diffusion restriction, or other signs of active myositis. All other muscles were

preserved. Echocardiography showed no cardiomyopathy. MR-angiography (MRA) did reveal a double aortic arch with a dominant right-sided arch and an incomplete left-sided arch (Fig. 3). At present he is a student and doing well.

Case Description 2

After normal pregnancy and delivery, patient 2 (male) was born to nonconsanguineous parents and presented at the age of 6 months with hypotonia. Despite physiotherapy, development of gross motor skills, including free sitting and standing, was delayed by several months. At the age of 17 months, occult spina bifida was noted, but no spinal cord abnormalities were seen on MRI. At 21 months, physical examination showed a length of 85 cm (−0.3 SD), a weight-to-length ratio of 10.6 kg/85 cm (−1.8 SD), and a head circumference of 49.3 cm (0 SD), notably underdeveloped musculature of all four limbs with mild hypotonia, externally rotated gait, and lumbar hyperlordosis. Creatine kinase (199 U/I) and aspartate transaminase (AST 64 U/I) levels were mildly elevated, while other liver enzymes remained within the reference range (ALT <40 U/I, LDH <400 U/L, and AP <300 U/L). Abdominal ultrasound did not show hepatosplenomegaly and musculoskeletal ultrasound, nerve conduction studies, and cardiac tests did not reveal abnormalities. The clinical presentation of generalized muscle atrophy without evident liver involvement had a wide differential diagnosis. It was most suspicious for selenoprotein-related myopathy, for which

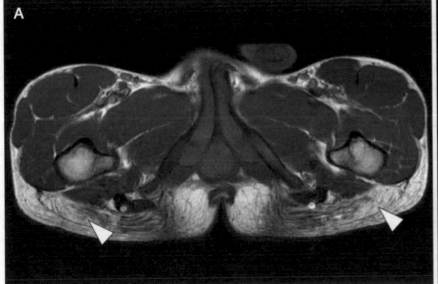
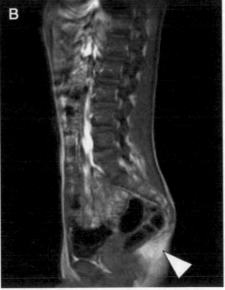

Fig. 2 T1-weighted MR images of patient 1 at age 17. The transverse section of the pelvis (**a**) and the sagittal section of the thorax, abdomen, and pelvis (**b**) demonstrated nearly complete bilateral replacement of the normal hypo-intense signal of gluteus maximus muscle with the hyperintense signal of fat (white arrowheads)

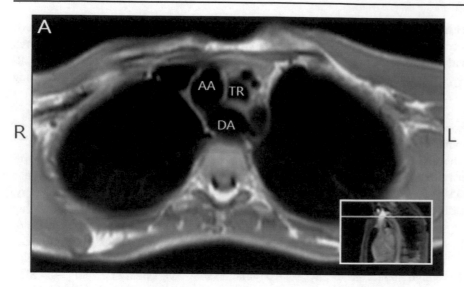
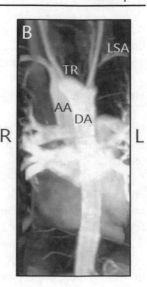

Fig. 3 Transverse MRI (**a**) and coronal MRI-angiography (**b**) in patient 1 showed a dominant right aortic arch and Kommerell diverticulum. The left subclavian artery (LSA) was not directly connected to the Kommerell diverticulum. Most likely an atypical duct previously connected the Kommerell diverticulum to the LSA. *TR* trachea, *AA* ascending aorta, *DA* descending aorta

muscle biopsies are often inconclusive. Therefore, a gene panel investigation into a broader range of disorders was performed.

Genetic and Enzymatic Evaluation

Investigation of 74 genes associated with distal myopathies revealed two missense mutations in the *GBE1* gene: c.[691+2T>C] splice donor variant (previously reported as pathogenic variant in severe GSD IV, Fernandez et al. 2010) and the same mutation as patient 1; c.[760A>G] p.[Thr254Ala] (previously reported, Said et al. 2016). As mentioned above, three pathogenicity prediction algorithms predicted T254A to be a disease-causing variant. The activity of GBE1 in red and white blood cells was severely reduced (5–10% of normal). No muscle biopsy was performed because genetic and enzymatic methods had already confirmed the diagnosis. Although laboratory and radiological findings did not suggest liver involvement, a continuous glucose monitoring was performed to rule out the possibility of unnoticed hypoglycemia. No hypoglycemic events occurred during 34 h, and glucose levels remained above 3.7 mmol/L during an 8-h overnight fast. At present, the patient is aged 3 years, no hypoglycemic events have occurred thus far, and he receives a normal diet. He still suffers from hypotonia, but motor skill development progresses, CK (148 U/L) and AST (35 U/L) values remain within the reference range, and weight-to-length ratio normalizes (15.7 kg/103.8 cm, −0.95 SD).

Discussion

GSD IV is an autosomal recessive metabolic disorder, with an incidence of 1:600,000–1:800,000. Classically, five clinical subtypes have been recognized. However, the widely heterogeneous presentations, varying in age of onset and affected organ systems, do not all fit well into these subtypes (Burrow et al. 2006). The patients here described presented with generalized hypotonia and myopathy and could be classified as presentations of the childhood neuromuscular subtype (Magoulas and El-Hattab 2013) with little (patient 1) to no (patient 2) involvement of the liver and a mild clinical course. However, fasting intolerance and decreased glycogenolytic capacity as observed and quantified in patient 1 have not been reported previously in this subtype. Indeed, hypoglycemia is rarely observed in GSD IV and only in the context of liver failure. This shows that the clinical spectrum of GSD IV is ever expanding and will likely further expand in the current age of genetic testing.

The severity of GSD IV phenotypes has been correlated to residual glycogen-branching enzyme activity, with null mutations leading to severe perinatal and congenital subtypes. However, it remains largely unclear how milder, biallelic mutations relate to organ involvement and disease progression (Magoulas and El-Hattab 2013). The c.[1063C>T]; p.[Arg355Cys] missense mutation identified in patient 1 has not been reported previously. It concerns a highly conserved (Fig. S1 in Supplementary Material)

arginine residue located in the catalytic core and has high predicted impact on protein function. The c.[691+2T>C] mutation identified in patient 2 affects a consensus splicing site and was previously described in a patient with congenital neuromuscular subtype and 20% residual enzyme activity in fibroblasts (Fernandez et al. 2010). The c.[760A>G] p.[Thr254Ala] mutation found in both our patients has recently been identified in one other patient with a mild classic hepatic subtype and >25% residual enzyme activity in fibroblasts (Said et al. 2016). When compared to these patients with similar genotypes, residual enzyme activity in our patients (patient 1: undetectable; patient 2: 5–10%) was remarkably low. Besides, patients reported in the literature with comparable childhood neuromuscular phenotypes typically had >10% residual activity in fibroblasts (Magoulas et al. 2012). This discrepancy might well be caused by the use of blood cells in our enzyme activity tests versus fibroblasts in most other reports, as residual activity can vary between cell types within the same individual (Li et al. 2010). In summary, both our patients with predominant muscular phenotypes have one unique mutation that has high predicted impact on protein function and share the milder c.[760A>G] p.[Thr254Ala] mutation previously identified in a patient with a predominant hepatic phenotype. This shows that it remains difficult to predict organ involvement based on genotype alone and suggests that other genetic or environmental factors also play a role.

The muscle MRI of patient 1 showed replacement of muscle with connective and adipose tissue in the gluteus maximus muscles. Although cardiomyopathy is a common finding in GSD IV, echocardiographic evaluation of our patient did not reveal this. However, MRA showed a double aortic arch, an unusual finding in the general population (estimated incidence 1:1,000–1:10,000). The co-occurrence of double aortic arch and GSD IV could be coincidental, but indications exist that *GBE1* mutations can modify structural cardiac development. First, Lee et al. (2011) showed abnormal cardiac development in a $GBE1^{-/-}$ mouse model. Second, double aortic arch has been reported in other storage disorders, including GSD II (Akalin et al. 2000) and mucopolysaccharidosis (Slepov and Chumakov 1997). Further investigations are needed into the possible correlation between *GBE1* mutations and structural cardiac abnormalities and into the possibility of these two conditions co-existing, independent of each other.

No polyglucosan bodies or other histopathological findings suggestive of GSD IV could be identified in the muscle biopsy of patient 1, even upon re-examination after the genetic diagnosis. A review of the literature revealed that the absence of polyglucosan bodies in biopsies from patients with GBE1 dysfunction is very rare

(Supplementary Table 2 in Supplementary Material). Out of 60 patients with GSD IV, only 1 patient did not have histopathological findings indicative of abnormal glycogen storage. Upon intensive re-examination of this patient's muscle biopsy after genetic diagnosis, sporadic polyglucosan bodies could be identified (Ravenscroft et al. 2013). Out of 24 patients with adult polyglucosan body disease, two patients did not have polyglucosan bodies in muscle biopsies (Colombo et al. 2015). Importantly, the literature might underestimate the percentage of GSD IV patients without polyglucosan bodies, because histopathological findings are key to the diagnosis when no (untargeted) genetic methods are available.

In conclusion, we present two patients with a similar neuromuscular presentation of GSD IV but with strikingly different diagnostic gaps: 17 years in patient 1 and 2 years in patient 2. Their cases illustrate the value of early genetic testing for rare genetic disorders. Genetic testing was especially helpful in patient 1, in which typical histopathological findings were absent from the muscle biopsy. However, genetic testing does have limitations including (1) false negatives due to low sequencing coverage or exclusion of disease-causing regions and (2) diagnostic dilemmas arising from variants of uncertain significance (Reid et al. 2016). Therefore, genetic testing should always be preceded by a thorough clinical workup and complemented by biochemical evaluations.

Synopsis

Our recent diagnoses of GSD IV in two patients with hypotonia and delayed development of gross motor skills further expand the clinical phenotype of GSD IV and demonstrate the value of early genetic testing in the diagnostic procedure of unresolved neuromuscular disorders.

Details of the Contributions of Individual Authors

IFS and GV drafted the manuscript and designed the figures with support of SF GV is the metabolic pediatrician of patient 1. GCK is the pediatric neurologist of patient 2. HHH interpreted the stable isotope fasting test in patient 1. LP is the clinical neurologist of patient 1. DD executed the genetic diagnostics in patient 1. JMPJB is the pediatric cardiologist who interpreted the echocardiography and MRI-angiography in patient 1. SB executed the genetic diagnostics in patient 2. All authors revised the manuscript.

Competing Interest Statement

The authors declare they have no conflicts of interest.

Ethics Approval and Patient Consent Statement

No ethics approval or patient consent was required for the presented findings.

References

Akalin F, Alper G, Oztunç F, Kotiloğlu E, Turan S (2000) A case of glycogen storage disease type II with double aortic arch. Acta Paediatr 89(7):884–886

Burrow TA, Hopkin RJ, Bove KE et al (2006) Non-lethal congenital hypotonia due to glycogen storage disease type IV. Am J Med Genet A 140:878–882

Choi M, Scholl UI, Ji W (2009) Genetic diagnosis by whole exome capture and massively parallel DNA sequencing. Proc Natl Acad Sci U S A 106(45):19096–19101

Colombo I, Pagliarani S, Testolin S et al (2015) Adult polyglucosan body disease: clinical and histological heterogeneity of a large Italian family. Neuromuscul Disord 25:423–428

Fernandez C, Halbert C, De Paula AM et al (2010) Non-lethal neonatal neuromuscular variant of glycogenosis type IV with novel GBE1 mutations. Muscle Nerve 41:269–271

Klein CJ (2013) Adult polyglucosan body disease. In: Pagon RA, Adam MP, Bird TD, Dolan CR, Fong CT, Smith RJ et al (eds) GeneReviews. University of Washington, Seattle. https://www.ncbi.nlm.nih.gov/books/NBK5300/. Retrieved 1 Dec 2017

Lee YC, Chang CJ, Bali D, Chen YT, Yan YT (2011) Glycogen-branching enzyme deficiency leads to abnormal cardiac development: novel insights into glycogen storage disease IV. Hum Mol Genet 20(3):455–456

Li S, Chen C, Goldstein J et al (2010) Glycogen storage disease type IV: novel mutations and molecular characterization of a heterogeneous disorder. J Inherit Metab Dis 33(3):S83–S90

Magoulas PL, El-Hattab AW (2013) Glycogen storage disease type IV. In: Pagon RA, Adam MP, Bird TD, Dolan CR, Fong CT, Smith RJ et al (eds) GeneReviews. University of Washington, Seattle. https://www.ncbi.nlm.nih.gov/books/NBK115333/. Retrieved 1 Dec 2017

Magoulas PL, El-Hattab AW, Angshumoy R, Bali DS, Finegold MJ, Craigen WJ (2012) Diffuse reticuloendothelial system involvement in type IV glycogen storage disease with a novel GBE1 mutation: a case report and review. Hum Pathol 43:943–951

Moses SW, Parvari R (2002) The variable presentations of glycogen storage disease type IV. Curr Mol Med 2(2):177–188

Ravenscroft G, Thompson EM, Todd EJ et al (2013) Whole exome sequencing in foetal akinesia expands the genotype-phenotype spectrum of GBE1 glycogen storage disease mutations. Neuromuscul Disord 23:165–169

Reid ES, Papandreou A, Drury S et al (2016) Advantages and pitfalls of an extended gene panel for investigating complex neuro-metabolic phenotypes. Brain 139:2844–2854

Said SM, Murphree MI, Mounajjed T, El-Youssef M, Zhang L (2016) A novel GBE1 gene variant in a child with glycogen storage disease type IV. Hum Pathol 54:152–156

Slepov AK, Chumakov LF (1997) Co-occurrence of double aortic arch with mucopolysaccharidosis in an infant. Klin Khir 7–8:105

JIMD Reports
DOI 10.1007/8904_2018_147

RESEARCH REPORT

A Hemizygous Deletion Within the *PGK1* Gene in Males with PGK1 Deficiency

Andrea Medrano Behlmann · Namita A. Goyal ·
Xiaoyu Yang · Ping H. Chen · Arunkanth Ankala

Received: 08 June 2018 /Revised: 24 August 2018 /Accepted: 25 September 2018 /Published online: 21 December 2018
© Society for the Study of Inborn Errors of Metabolism (SSIEM) 2018

Abstract Phosphoglycerate kinase-1 (PGK1) deficiency is a rare X-linked disorder caused by pathogenic variants in the *PGK1* gene. Complete loss-of-function variants have not been reported in this gene, indicating that residual enzyme function is critical for viability in males. Therefore, copy number variants (CNVs) that include single exon or multiple exon deletions or duplications are generally not expected in individuals with PGK1 deficiency. Here we describe a 64-year-old male presenting with a family history (three additional affected males) and a personal history of childhood-onset metabolic myopathy that involves episodes of muscle pain, stiffness after activity, exercise intolerance, and myoglobinuria after exertion. Biochemical analysis on a muscle biopsy indicated significantly reduced activity (15% compared to normal) for phosphoglycerate kinase (PGK1), a glycolytic enzyme encoded by *PGK1*. A diagnosis of PGK1 deficiency was established by molecular analysis which detected an approximately 886 kb deletion involving the polyadenylation site in the 3′UTR of the *PGK1* gene. RNA analysis showed significantly reduced *PGK1* transcript levels (30% compared to normal). This is the first deletion reported in the *PGK1* gene and is the first pathogenic variant involving the 3′UTR polyadenylation site of this gene. Our report emphasizes the role of 3′UTR variants in human disorders and underscores the need for exploring noncoding regions of disease-associated genes when seeking a molecular diagnosis.

Introduction

Phosphoglycerate kinase-1 (PGK1) deficiency (MIM# 300653) is a rare X-linked disorder that is clinically heterogeneous and presents with hemolytic anemia, muscular defects, and neurological dysfunction. The disease exists in two major forms: the hemolytic subtype, in which affected individuals have hereditary non-spherocytic hemolytic anemia (HNSA), and the myopathic form, characterized by progressive muscle weakness, pain, and cramping (Beutler 2007). Both forms can be accompanied by intellectual disability or other neurological manifestations (Fermo et al. 2012).

PGK1 deficiency is caused by pathogenic variants in the *PGK1* gene. *PGK1* encodes a phosphoglycerate kinase (EC.2.7.2.3) that catalyzes a critical ATP-generating step of glycolysis. A single pathogenic variant in a hemizygous copy of the *PGK1* gene causes disease in males; female carriers are typically asymptomatic or demonstrate chronic, mild hemolytic anemia (Valentine et al. 1968). At least 25 different *PGK1* pathogenic variants, all of which are

Andrea Medrano Behlmann and Namita A. Goyal contributed equally to this work.

Communicated by: Avihu Boneh

Electronic supplementary material: The online version of this chapter (https://doi.org/10.1007/8904_2018_147) contains supplementary material, which is available to authorized users.

A. M. Behlmann · A. Ankala (✉)
Department of Human Genetics, Emory University School of Medicine, Atlanta, GA, USA
e-mail: aankala@emory.edu

N. A. Goyal
Department of Neurology, University of California, Irvine, CA, USA

X. Yang · P. H. Chen
Department of Cell Biology, Emory University School of Medicine, Atlanta, GA, USA

A. Ankala
EGL Genetic Diagnostics LLC, Tucker, GA, USA

sequence variants, have been reported in the literature. These include 16 missense variants, 2 small (less than 5 basepairs) deletions within exons, and 4 splice site variants, all of which are expected to reduce, but not completely abolish, expression levels, stability, or enzymatic efficiency of the PGK1 protein (Stenson et al. 2017). Complete loss-of-function variants have not been reported in this gene, indicating that residual enzyme function is critical for viability in males (Chiarelli et al. 2012; Pey et al. 2014). Therefore, copy number variants (CNVs) that include single exon or multiple exon deletions or duplications are generally not expected in patients with PGK1 deficiency. Here we report a familial PGK1 deficiency caused by a novel 886 kb deletion located downstream of the translation termination site and involving the 3′UTR polyadenylation (poly-A) sequence; the entire *PGK1* coding region is otherwise intact. This is the first pathogenic CNV and the first 3′UTR variant ever reported in *PGK1*.

Clinical Report

A 64-year-old Caucasian male presented with a childhood-onset metabolic myopathy characterized by episodes of muscle pain, muscle stiffness, exercise intolerance, and myoglobinuria after activity. One episode of rhabdomyolysis occurred during the fifth decade of life. The patient is asymptomatic at rest and does not require assistance with daily activities or assistive devices for mobility, but rests between activities that require exertion. Creatine kinase (CK) levels have reportedly been elevated since childhood and ranged from 600 to 7,000 U/L for the past year. He has mild proximal weakness of shoulder girdle and hip girdle muscles. EMG findings indicated a nonirritable myopathy. Dried blood spot test showed normal acid alpha-glucosidase level arguing against Pompe disease. Muscle biopsy showed normal routine histology, arguing against a dystrophic myopathy or a mitochondrial myopathy.

Given the concern for a metabolic myopathy, a comprehensive biochemical evaluation of the patient's muscle tissue was performed. Biochemical analysis of a muscle biopsy revealed significant deficiency of PGK1 enzyme activity (18 μmol/min/g tissue compared to a normal reference mean of 116.5 μmol/min/g; reference range of 48–184), indicating a possible diagnosis of PGK1 deficiency. Biochemical analysis of all enzyme levels in the myoglobinuria profile panel including myophosphorylase, phosphorylase b kinase, phosphofructokinase, phosphoglycerate mutase, carnitine palmitoyltransferase, lactate dehydrogenase, myoadenylate deaminase was normal. This residual PGK1 activity of 15% is comparable to those reported in individuals with a clinical diagnosis of PGK1 deficiency (Chiarelli et al. 2012). Congruent myopathic

symptoms were noted in the patient's maternal uncle, brother, and sister's son, consistent with an X-linked disorder (Fig. 1a). No history of anemia or neurological dysfunction was noted in the proband or other affected family members.

Molecular Analysis and RNA Quantification

PGK1 Sanger sequencing and deletion/duplication analysis by array CGH were performed at EGL Genetics (Tucker, GA, USA), a CAP and CLIA-certified clinical laboratory. Deletion breakpoint mapping analysis was performed using sequence-specific primers as described previously (Ankala et al. 2012). RNA was isolated from peripheral blood and analyzed by RT-PCR. All samples were run in triplicate and products were visualized on an agarose gel. RNA quantification and relative *PGK1* RNA expression (normalized to β-actin) were performed with imaging software (Image Studio Lite, version 3.1; Li-Cor Biosciences, Lincoln, Nebraska, USA) according to the manufacturer's instructions.

Results

Sequence analysis of the coding region and flanking intronic sequences of *PGK1* did not detect any sequence variants (benign, pathogenic, or otherwise). Subsequently, analysis for intragenic deletions or duplications was performed using array CGH. No CNVs were detected within the protein-coding region of the *PGK1* gene; however, an 886 kb deletion with genomic breakpoints at nucleotide positions g.77,381,971 and g.78,268,131 (hg19 reference; X chromosome; ClinVar accession number SCV000678240) and located approximately 600 bp downstream of the translation termination site of the *PGK1* gene was detected (Fig. 1b, c). This deletion encompasses the terminal portion of the 3′UTR and includes the poly-A signal sequence (ATTAAA) of the gene (Thierry-Mieg and Thierry-Mieg 2006). It also includes five additional genes, *TAF9B, CYSLTR1, ZCCHC5, LPAR4*, and *P2RY10*, none of which have been associated with human diseases. A deletion involving this region of the human genome has not been reported in the general population (MacDonald et al. 2014) or in individuals with disease (Stenson et al. 2003). The proband's affected brother was also found to carry this deletion (Fig. 2a). Quantitative analysis of RNA extracted from the peripheral blood sample of the affected brothers showed significantly reduced (37–40%) transcript levels of *PGK1* when compared to that of a gender-matched unaffected control (Fig. 2b). No other family members were available for testing. While the segregation analysis shown here is limited, all other lines of evidence including

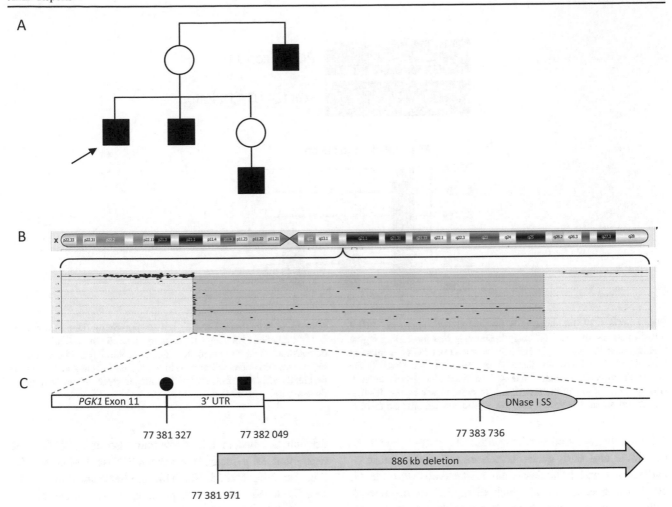

Fig. 1 (**a**) The proband (arrow) reports that his maternal uncle, brother, and sister's son share similar myopathic symptoms (black squares), consistent with an X-linked disorder. (**b**) Deletion and duplication analysis by CGH detected an 866 kb deletion in the noncoding region downstream of *PGK1*. (**c**) The 5′ breakpoint of the deletion occurs 600 bp downstream of the PGK1 translation termination codon (black circle). The deletion (gray arrow) encompasses a portion of the 3′UTR, including the polyadenylation site (ATTAAA; black square) and a DNase sensitive site (DNase I SS; gray oval) that may act as a *PGK1* transcription regulatory element. Numbers indicate genomic location of labeled sites (hg19, chromosome X). Genetic elements are not to scale

biochemical (reduced enzyme activity), molecular (reduced transcript levels), population data (absent in population), and family history (X-linked inheritance) suggest that the observed deletion is potentially pathogenic.

Discussion

After a comprehensive analysis involving clinical evaluation, enzyme activity assays on muscle biopsy, molecular investigation of genomic DNA, and RNA quantitation, we establish a diagnosis of PGK1 deficiency in a 64-year-old male with a childhood-onset metabolic myopathy. We report the first pathogenic variant within the 3′UTR of the *PGK1* gene: an 886 kb deletion involving the poly-A site. Our report of the first pathogenic CNV within the *PGK1* gene expands the mutation spectrum of the gene and establishes the clinical utility of deletion/duplication

analysis for PGK1 deficiency as a follow-up test for individuals with a clinical diagnosis of PGK1 deficiency but negative sequencing results.

3′UTRs are known to contain important sequence elements that collectively determine the fate of mRNA, from its post-transcriptional modifications, stability, and half-life to its export from the nucleus and successful translation into a full-length polypeptide. An important component of this region is the poly-A signal sequence, which is critical for proper transcription termination, post-transcriptional pre-mRNA cleavage, and subsequent placement of the poly-A tail (Chen et al. 2006). Several variants that disrupt this sequence have been associated with disease. These include single nucleotide variants (SNVs) in the poly-A hexamer of the *FOXP3* gene that causes IPEX syndrome (Bennett et al. 2001) and of the *IL2RG* gene that causes severe combined immunodeficiency syndrome (SCID; Hsu et al. 2009).

A

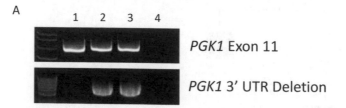

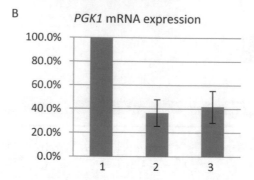

Fig. 2 *PGK1* 3′UTR deletion is associated with decreased *PGK1* mRNA expression. (**a**) PCR analysis showing that the coding region (gel image at the top) of the last exon (exon 11) of *PGK1* is intact in (lane 1) a control sample, (lane 2) the proband, and (lane 3) the proband's affected brother. Lane 4 is a blank (no DNA) control. Breakpoint-junction primers designed to amplify across the deletion (intact control sample would not give a product) demonstrate that the

affected brothers (lanes 2 and 3), but not the control (lane 1), carry the 3′ UTR deletion (gel image at the bottom). (**b**) Relative RNA analysis demonstrates that compared to a normal control (1), *PGK1* mRNA expression was decreased to 37% in the proband (2) and to 42% in the proband's affected brother (3). Percentages represent an average of three separate experiments

Additionally, deletion variants within the poly-A signals of the *HBA2* and *HBB* genes have been reported to cause α-thalassemia and β⁺-thalassemia, respectively (Prior et al. 2007; Rund et al. 1992). Such disruption of the poly-A signal has been reported to result in read-through transcripts extending past the normal poly-A cleavage site, resulting in aberrant transcription termination and RNA splicing and processing (Rund et al. 1992). Although these longer and abnormal transcripts are reported as unstable and likely targeted by nonsense mediated decay (Chen et al. 2006), they are also translatable in vivo and can contribute to residual protein expression (Rund et al. 1992). This likely explains the residual PGK1 enzyme activity and metabolic myopathy in our study individuals.

Variants outside the poly-A signal sequence have also been identified as causative of disease. These include the 13 bp deletion and the c.*32A>C variant in the 3′UTR of the β-globin mRNA (*HBB* gene) which result in thalassemia by affecting nuclear processing of the mRNA or by decreasing mRNA stability, respectively (Bilenoglu et al. 2002; Hino et al. 2012). Alternatively, similar variants that disrupt 3′UTR sequences may alter recruitment of *trans*-acting factors which regulate gene expression or modify the 3′UTR secondary structure, thereby leading to disease (Chen et al. 2006). Gene expression (temporal and/or spatial) may also be altered by variants that disrupt chromosomal structure around a gene and/or of the *cis*-acting long-range regulatory elements (reviewed in Maston et al. 2006). Similarly, the

deletion detected in this study may also alter *PGK1* gene expression as it includes a known DNase I sensitive site (Fig. 1c; Riley et al. 1991). This site has been shown to be specific to the actively expressing *PGK1* allele and is suggested to play a role as a regulatory element in mediating chromatin configuration around the *PGK1* gene and in regulating its expression. The possible mechanisms (of position effect) by which this potential regulatory element may alter *PGK1* gene expression are illustrated in the supplementary data (Fig. S1).

For a metabolic disease like PGK1 deficiency that is very rare and has a wide clinical spectrum that ranges from death in early childhood to being asymptomatic (Beutler 2007), making a molecular diagnosis and understanding the genotype–phenotype correlation are important. Given the high clinical variability, it is highly likely that the disease in general is underdiagnosed. In the current study, the negative sequencing result for *PGK1*, an X-linked gene (with only one copy in a male) would have likely ruled out a deletion and potentially evaded the diagnosis, had the subsequent CNV analysis not been performed. Therefore, it is critical that a comprehensive genetic evaluation (that includes SNV and CNV analysis) be made, especially when there is a strong clinical suspicion of a genetic disorder. Occasionally, mosaicism for CNVs has been reported in males with a milder presentation of an otherwise lethal X-linked disorder (Maddalena et al. 1988), which further emphasizes the need for complete genetic analysis.

Our findings further demonstrate the importance of investigating the noncoding regions of the genome. The promoter region, protein-coding exons, noncoding exons that comprise the 5′ and 3′ untranslated regions (UTRs), and interspersing introns together constitute the basic structure of a functional eukaryotic gene. However, given the lack of complete understanding of the sequence context of each individual gene and transcript in the human genome, molecular diagnostics is most often confined to variants within the protein-coding region. Currently, CNVs and SNVs within these noncoding and regulatory regions, that potentially modify gene expression and cause diseases, typically escape most routine molecular diagnostic tests. However, as investigation of the roles of 5′ and 3′ UTRs and other regulatory elements continues, and reports of disease-causing variants within these regions emerge (Ma et al. 2015), the need for interrogating these regions will increase. The rapidly reducing costs of sequencing are expected to further facilitate this, thereby allowing for increased clinical diagnostic yield.

Synopsis

This report of a PGK1 deficiency case caused by a novel hemizygous deletion in the *PGK1* gene demonstrates the need to include exon level copy number analysis in the diagnostic workup to fully exclude this disorder.

Author Contributions

Andrea Behlmann contributed to analysis and interpretation of data and drafted the chapter.

Namita Goyal contributed to conception and design and revised it critically.

Xiaoyu Yang contributed to conception and design and drafted the chapter.

Ping Chen contributed to analysis and interpretation of data and revised it critically.

Arunkanth Ankala contributed to conception and design and revised it critically and is the Guarantor for the study.

Competing Interest

Andrea Behlmann, Namita Goyal, Xiaoyu Yang, and Ping Chen declare no conflict of interest. Arunkanth Ankala is employed by Emory University and is a laboratory director at EGL Genetic Diagnostics, LLC, a clinical genetics laboratory which performs testing described in this paper.

Funding

None.

Ethics Approval/Patient Consent

No individually identifiable patient information is used.

Animal Usage

None.

References

Ankala A, Kohn JN, Hegde A, Meka A, Ephrem CL, Askree SH et al (2012) Aberrant firing of replication origins potentially explains intragenic nonrecurrent rearrangements within genes, including the human DMD gene. Genome Res 22(1):25–34. https://doi.org/10.1101/gr.123463.111

Bennett CL, Brunkow ME, Ramsdell F, O'Briant KC, Zhu Q, Fuleihan RL et al (2001) A rare polyadenylation signal mutation of the FOXP3 gene (AAUAAA–>AAUGAA) leads to the IPEX syndrome. Immunogenetics 53(6):435–439. https://doi.org/10.1007/s002510100358

Beutler E (2007) PGK deficiency. Br J Haematol 136(1):3–11. https://doi.org/10.1111/j.1365-2141.2006.06351.x

Bilenoglu O, Basak AN, Russell JE (2002) A 3′UTR mutation affects beta-globin expression without altering the stability of its fully processed mRNA. Br J Haematol 119(4):1106–1114

Chen JM, Ferec C, Cooper DN (2006) A systematic analysis of disease-associated variants in the 3′ regulatory regions of human protein-coding genes II: the importance of mRNA secondary structure in assessing the functionality of 3′ UTR variants. Hum Genet 120(3):301–333. https://doi.org/10.1007/s00439-006-0218-x

Chiarelli LR, Morera SM, Bianchi P, Fermo E, Zanella A, Galizzi A, Valentini G (2012) Molecular insights on pathogenic effects of mutations causing phosphoglycerate kinase deficiency. PLoS One 7(2):e32065. https://doi.org/10.1371/journal.ponc.0032065

Fermo E, Bianchi P, Chiarelli LR, Maggi M, Mandara GM, Vercellati C et al (2012) A new variant of phosphoglycerate kinase deficiency (p.I371K) with multiple tissue involvement: molecular and functional characterization. Mol Genet Metab 106(4):455–461. https://doi.org/10.1016/j.ymgme.2012.05.015

Hino M, Yamashiro Y, Hattori Y, Ito H, Nitta T, Adhiyanto C et al (2012) Identification of a novel mutation in the beta-globin gene 3′ untranslated region [+1,506 (A>C)] in a Japanese male with a heterozygous beta-thalassemia phenotype. Hemoglobin 36(2):170–176. https://doi.org/10.3109/03630269.2011.647186

Hsu AP, Fleisher TA, Niemela JE (2009) Mutation analysis in primary immunodeficiency diseases: case studies. Curr Opin Allergy Clin Immunol 9(6):517–524. https://doi.org/10.1097/ACI.0-b013e3283328f59

Ma M, Ru Y, Chuang LS, Hsu NY, Shi LS, Hakenberg J et al (2015) Disease-associated variants in different categories of disease located in distinct regulatory elements. BMC Genomics 16(Suppl 8):S3. https://doi.org/10.1186/1471-2164-16-S8-S3

MacDonald JR, Ziman R, Yuen RK, Feuk L, Scherer SW (2014) The Database of Genomic Variants: a curated collection of structural variation in the human genome. Nucleic Acids Res 42(Database issue):D986–D992. https://doi.org/10.1093/nar/gkt958

Maddalena A, Sosnoski DM, Berry GT, Nussbaum RL (1988) Mosaicism for an intragenic deletion in a boy with mild ornithine transcarbamylase deficiency. N Engl J Med 319(15):999–1003. https://doi.org/10.1056/NEJM198810133191507

Maston GA, Evans SK, Green MR (2006) Transcriptional regulatory elements in the human genome. Annu Rev Genomics Hum Genet 7:29–59. https://doi.org/10.1146/annurev.genom.7.080505.115623

Pey AL, Maggi M, Valentini G (2014) Insights into human phosphoglycerate kinase 1 deficiency as a conformational disease from biochemical, biophysical, and in vitro expression analyses. J Inherit Metab Dis 37(6):909–916. https://doi.org/10.1007/s10545-014-9721-8

Prior JF, Lim E, Lingam N, Raven JL, Finlayson J (2007) A moderately severe alpha-thalassemia condition resulting from a combination of the alpha2 polyadenylation signal (AATAAA–> AATA- -) mutation and a 3.7 Kb alpha gene deletion in an Australian family. Hemoglobin 31(2):173–177. https://doi.org/10.1080/03630260701288997

Riley DE, Goldman MA, Gartler SM (1991) Nucleotide sequence of the 3′ nuclease-sensitive region of the human phosphoglycerate kinase 1 (PGK1) gene. Genomics 11(1):212–214

Rund D, Dowling C, Najjar K, Rachmilewitz EA, Kazazian HH Jr, Oppenheim A (1992) Two mutations in the beta-globin polyadenylylation signal reveal extended transcripts and new RNA polyadenylylation sites. Proc Natl Acad Sci U S A 89(10):4324–4328

Stenson PD, Ball EV, Mort M, Phillips AD, Shiel JA, Thomas NS et al (2003) Human Gene Mutation Database (HGMD): 2003 update. Hum Mutat 21(6):577–581. https://doi.org/10.1002/humu.10212

Stenson PD, Mort M, Ball EV, Evans K, Hayden M, Heywood S et al (2017) The Human Gene Mutation Database: towards a comprehensive repository of inherited mutation data for medical research, genetic diagnosis and next-generation sequencing studies. Hum Genet 136(6):665–677. https://doi.org/10.1007/s00439-017-1779-6

Thierry-Mieg D, Thierry-Mieg J (2006) AceView: a comprehensive cDNA-supported gene and transcripts annotation. Genome Biol 7(Suppl 1):S12.11–S12.14. https://doi.org/10.1186/gb-2006-7-s1-s12

Valentine WN, Hsieh HS, Paglia DE, Anderson HM, Baughan MA, Jaffe ER, Garson OM (1968) Hereditary hemolytic anemia: association with phosphoglycerate kinase deficiency in erythrocytes and leukocytes. Trans Assoc Am Phys 81:49–65

Printed in the United States
By Bookmasters